D1794785

Establishing Health Priorities
in the Developing World

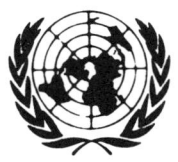

Published by:
Adams Publishing Group, Ltd., 1988
P.O. Box 263, Prudential Center,
Boston, MA.

Under the auspices of
United Nations Development Programme.

Establishing Health Priorities in the Developing World

Julia A. Walsh, M.D., D.T.P.H.*

Harvard School of Public Health
Boston, Massachusetts

United Nations Development Programme

Division for Global and Interregional Programmes
One United Nations Plaza
New York, New York 10017

SOURCES: The information and opinions expressed in this publication derive from a review of the references cited plus a general background literature review. In addition, the author has discussed many of the topics with experts in various aspects of tropical health and research at the World Health Organization, World Bank, and a variety of academic institutions. The views expressed in this monograph are those of the author and other experts in the field and do not necessarily reflect those of the United Nations Development Programme.

Preface

The United Nations Development Programme, Divison for Global and Interregional Programmes, commissioned this monograph to stimulate a dialogue among national and international agencies, universities (including schools of public administration, economics, medicine and public health), and individuals committed to improving the health of people living in developing countries. By addressing such topics as the status of health, scientific and technological health developments, and strategies and interventions for improving health, this monograph intends to facilitate information exchange and the decision-making process, leading to the judicious allocation of scarce financial resources for health.

The people involved in this process—specifically, the ministers of finance, planning and health, and international agency officials—may wish to consider the methodology for priority-setting discussed herein.

The publication of this monograph coincides with two important international events, namely:

A. The creation of the International Commission on Health Research for Development, of which the main objective is to improve health in the developing world by enlarging research activities, speeding up the application of research results, and mobilizing resources for this purpose. The monograph will serve as a major input to the Commission's work; and

B. The third high-level policy meeting on the subject of "Protecting the World's Children" (Bellagion III) to be held in Talloires, France, March 10-12, 1988. The Bellagio III Conference will review progress made in immunization and other health interventions affecting the health of children, and consider what still must be done to sustain vaccine and other research activities during the remainder of this century.

Since changes occur rapidly in the field as a result of research developments, epidemics, and varying social and economic status, the UNDP plans to update this publication in three or four years.

Individuals from the UNDP and many other United Nations Agencies have provided valuable input through their generous consideration and comments on earlier drafts and valuable time in discussion. The World Health Organization, UNICEF, and the World Bank have been particularly helpful. Academicians, health planners, and officials of other multilateral, bilateral, and non-governmental agencies have also lent their time and interest to this endeavour.

Timothy Rothermel
Director
Division for Global and Interregional
Programmes
United Nations Development Programme
March 1988

Acknowledgment

This monograph on setting health priorities in the developing world was initiated through discussions with Frank Hartvelt from the Division for Global and Interregional Programmes, of the United Nations Development Programme. His valuable comments and encouragement forged a strong foundation for this effort. Others who donated their time and consideration to this project include numerous individuals: from the World Health Organization (T. Godal, R. Cook, A. Petros-Barvazian, R. Henderson, A. Creese, A. Pio, G. Torigiani, R. Mansourian, J. Martin, A. Hammad, M. Merson, P. Rosenfield),

from the United Nations Development Programme, (M. Sachs),

from academic institutions such as Harvard School of Public Health (L. Chen, D. Bell, R. Cash, among others), the Prince Leopold Institute for Tropical Diseases, Belgium (H. Van Baelen, P. Mercenier), the Royal Tropical Institute, Amsterdam (A. Muller),

and from other agencies: K. Edstrom and V. Ramalingaswami (UNICEF), A. Measham and D. Jamison (World Bank), K.S. Warren (The Rockefeller Foundation), W. Stinson (PRICOR), among others.

I wish to express my deep appreciation for their time and efforts on behalf of this project.

Finally, to Ann Adams of Adams Publishing Group, Ltd., for immeasurable assistance in the design and production of this book.

Julia A. Walsh, M.D., D.T.P.H.
Harvard School of Public Health
Boston, MA

About the Author

Julia A. Walsh is a physician who has trained in infectious diseases and tropical public health at New York University School of Medicine, University of California, San Francisco, and at the London School of Hygiene and Tropical Medicine. She has worked extensively in Kenya, India, Thailand, Mexico, Belize, Philippines, Egypt, and Nepal on studies involving epidemiologic operations, and health services research and on policy and program development. She is currently an Assistant Professor at Harvard Medical School in the Department of Medicine, Division of Infectious Diseases, and Associate Physician at the Brigham and Women's Hospital, Boston, Massachusetts. At the Harvard School of Public Health, she teaches health care planning and infectious disease epidemiology in developing countries and directs a course on public health issues of vaccines. She has worked as a consultant for the United Nations Development Programme, The Rockefeller Foundation, United States Agency for International Development, World Health Organization, and many other organizations. Among her publications, she has recently edited two books: *Strategies for Primary Health Care: Technologies Appropriate for the Control of Disease in the Developing World* with Dr. Kenneth S. Warren and *Good Health at Low Cost* with Dr. Kenneth S. Warren and Dr. Scott Halstead, Rockefeller Foundation. She is a practicing physician specializing in the care of infectious disease patients.

Contents

1 Establishing Priorities

Executive Summary

Balancing limited resources with needs for health improvement requires setting priorities. The status of health services and research, as well as societal, economic, and behavioral factors, all affect personal well-being.

The priorities for providing primary health care may differ from the priorities for research. For health services, the equitable, population-based provision of interventions of proven efficacy that are inexpensive, cost-effective, and technically feasible is paramount. These interventions must concentrate on those most in need. Health research, on the other hand, involves identifying barriers to good health, examining possible solutions, and then supporting laboratory studies and field trials. The research process involves a broad range of activities: biomedical research to develop better preventive or treatment methods; engineering improvements to simplify use and streamline operations and management; health systems evaluation; innovative financing schemes; methods for policy-making; to name a few. Simply stated, establishing priorities means carefully weighing the costs and potential benefits of the alternatives.

The process of prioritizing both for research and health services commences with an analysis of the major causes of morbidity and mortality. Local or national decision-makers use local and regional information, while international agencies use global estimates. For those major causes of ill health that have cost-effective control measures, research focuses on identifying better ways to utilize current measures. For conditions that lack adequate interventions (*i.e.*, current measures are inefficacious, costly, inconvenient, or associated with poor compliance), research concentrates on the development of new methods. Areas of research may include epidemiology, biotechnology, health systems analysis, policy-making, socio-economics, and so forth. Other factors affecting the selection of priorities include: assessment of the potential for the research to ultimately improve health, costs of research, capabilities, location of the research institutions, likelihood of successful outcomes, funding availability, and flexibility.

Setting priorities for health services implementation at the local level entails identification of the burden of illness, available interventions and cost-effectiveness, feasibility, ease of implementation, and likelihood of success.

Despite the declines in infant and child mortality rates, which have occurred in practically all countries of the world within the last 25 years, death of children under five years of age still accounts for the majority of deaths. Moreover, the causes of death among infants and children are among the leading causes of death for all ages. Respiratory infections, diseases of the circulatory system, low birth weight, diarrheal disease, and measles are the five most common causes. Injuries, malnutrition, neoplasms, malaria, and tetanus follow.

Several of these diseases or conditions are easily prevented and treated by currently available methods. Measles and tetanus, for example, are readily prevented by immunization; diarrheal disease is treated with oral rehydration therapy and preventive measures include handwashing, breast-feeding, and water and sanitation; respiratory infections are treated with antibiotics and prevented by breast-feeding; malaria is treated with drugs and prevented by control of human-vector contact. Nevertheless, a surprisingly substantial proportion of the world's population is without knowledge of, or access to, these control measures.

Health Research

The first goal of the *global* research agenda is to identify and test ways to improve use of known control measures. The second goal is to find new or better ones. Those opportunities thought to afford the greatest potential health benefits within the next several years are listed below. Applying the powerful new methods in biotechnology (genetic engineering) to develop new and improved vaccines, drugs, and diagnostic agents represents one of the greatest opportunities for global health advancement. Efforts in many of these areas are already under way, but increased investment would naturally hasten the achievement of the results. Of note, enormous global resources have already been committed to several important areas, such as Acquired Immune Deficiency Syndrome (AIDS) and cancer. Additional investments in these areas, particularly if they divert needed research funding from other important areas, such as child survival, would distort the *global* priorities. *Local* and *national* level priorities can be established using the same process outlined above, but may yield somewhat different results.

Programs to increase research in any of these areas must include the strengthening of institutions in the developing world, linkages among scientists, and training, in addition to the actual funding of studies. Each of the following research areas entails a range of research levels (basic, applied, epidemiologic, social, etc.) to ensure that the results rapidly traverse the journey from laboratory to village.

Priorities for future research

- *Application of the powerful biotechnology techniques* to develop new and improved vaccines, drugs, diagnostics, and vector control techniques for those diseases with the highest morbidity and mortality.

- *Identification of large field sites for epidemiologic studies,* field trials of present and future vaccines, drugs, diagnostics, other interventions, and evaluation of innovations in health care delivery systems. This task includes census and mapping of the population, preliminary assessment of risk factors, capacity building among institutions and individuals, and finally, study initiation.

- *Examination of the role of communications* and news media in health promotion, and training and development of new innovative uses of such media as radio, television, video, computer video, etc.

3

Health education is an effective tool for promoting health because it increases self-reliance.

• *Operations and health services research* that is particularly directed toward the efficient, population-based provision of control measures for the diseases of high priority. Such research stimulates a problem-solving attitude among all health workers and gradually enlarges the capacity of the health services to deal with an increasing array of conditions.

• *Improving the efficiency and functioning of management information systems,* including rapid assessment techniques. Evaluation and innovation of information systems could be considered operations research; however, it plays such a key role that it warrants specific attention.

Specific conditions requiring more research:

• *Acute Respiratory Infection.*   Requires (1) better preventive measures, such as vaccines, prophylaxis, environmental modification, increased breast-feeding; (2) better therapeutic case management using improved diagnostic agents and drug treatments; (3) more behavior and health education studies to improve effectiveness.

• *Low Birth Weight.*   Requires epidemiologic studies, development of interventions, and then evaluation and employment of results. These studies should specifically include study of maternal infection in pregnancy and its effect on the outcome of pregnancy for both the mother and infant. The cohort of mothers at high risk of maternal morbidity practically coincides with those at high risk for delivering low-birth-weight infants. Studies in this area will therefore benefit both mothers and infants.

• *Injury.*   Requires epidemiologic studies followed by development and testing of interventions.

• *Tuberculosis.*   Requires prevention and treatment through better vaccines and short-term drug therapy.

The application of research offers great opportunities for rapid improvements in child survival. Biotechnology, together with applied research to make available the new technologies and approaches as soon as possible, is the opportunity which seems to offer the greatest promise. The journey from laboratory to village should forge new international partnerships in research among scientists and field investigators of all countries. Research funding at the national and local level is a powerful tool for solving problems resulting from rapid expansion of the health system. Increasing local participation in research will lead to better deployment of the existing resources towards studies that can directly aid the decision-making process.

Health Services

Fortunately, many of the sicknesses affecting people in the developing world can be prevented. Vaccines, drugs, oral rehydration therapy, health education, water and sanitation, to name only a few, can significantly shorten the days of disability and decrease the risk of dying. Unfortunately, however, resources in the developing world are seriously limited and careful planning is required in order to most effectively and equitably use those resources to improve health. The planning of priorities for health services involves many of the same processes as the analysis used in setting research priorities: These include analysis of causes of burden of sickness, intervention strategies available, risk groups, and resources, among others.

High priority, efficacious interventions that are inexpensive, feasible, and capable of averting a substantial burden of sickness include: immunizations for measles, tetanus, whooping cough, and polio according to the schedule recommended by the Expanded Programme on Immunization (EPI); oral rehydration therapy; case-management of acute respiratory infections; malaria control; health education for personal hygiene and breast-feeding; vitamin A supplementation; and family planning. As the following measures become less expensive, they should also be considered: annual or semiannual treatment for worm infestations and filaria, typhoid vaccine, hepatitis B vaccine, and nutrition education. Depending on the diseases present locally, all or only some of these may be valuable and others may be added.

Access to health services has markedly improved, but their impact has been disappointing. Successful, sustained programs seem to emphasize good planning with setting of clear objectives and attainable targets; careful implementation based on a flexible problem-solving approach; a personnel policy that emphasizes training, supervision, and a people-oriented management style; sound financial policies, including partial cost recovery; and continuous monitoring and evaluation. The elements needed in a particular locale to improve health services requires study of the specific situation, but must certainly include attention to the underserved.

2 *Status of Health & Interventions*

Introduction

Establishing priorities for health research and implementation in the developing world, where the causes of ill health, death, and disability are numerous but the resources for health research and service are limited, is a difficult task. Although progress has been made in controlling many of the causes of ill health, inhabitants of the developing world still suffer a much greater burden of illness compared to citizens of industrialized countries, and many constraints remain.

Most of the countries of the world spend between 2% and 8% of their budgets on health (World Bank, 1987a). However, 50% or more of this budget may be committed to the maintenance of central hospitals and other institutions that are accessible only to a small proportion of the population. In addition to government expenditures, households may spend more than twice the total public expenditures, seeking health services in the private sector (World Bank, 1987b). Approximately 60% of all children presently have access to some kind of health facility, yet in many countries, fewer than 10% have received immunizations (Henderson, 1985; WHO, 1987).

Since the *Alma Ata Declaration* in 1978 focused attention on the importance of primary health care, governments have rapidly built peripheral health facilities for initial contact with the sick and for preventive measures. Nevertheless, in order for everyone to have adequate primary health care, efforts are required in three areas: (1) providing services where none exist, (2) improving the utilization of existing services, and (3) upgrading services to meet all the essential components of primary health care delivery. These essential components include: education concerning prevailing health problems and the methods of preventing and controlling them; promotion of food supply and proper nutrition; adequate supply of safe water and basic sanitation; maternal and child care services including family planning; immunization against the major infectious diseases; prevention and control of locally endemic diseases; appropriate treatment of common diseases and injuries; and provision of essential drugs (WHO-UNICEF, 1978).

Providing these components requires a major commitment of manpower, facilities, equipment, and finances, and the needs must be balanced against the shortage of resources available. Hence some difficult decisions must be made with respect to establishing reasonable priorities. The writers of the *Alma Ata Declaration* recognized these acute limitations when they stated:

The time has come for all levels of the health system to review critically their methods, techniques, equipment and drugs, with the aim of using only those technologies that have really proved their worth and can be afforded. National strategies should take into account socio-economic factors and policies, available resources, and the particular health problems and needs of the population with initial emphasis on the underserved.

The limitations on health *research* for prevention and/or cure of the causes of ill health in the developing world are several. The majority of public and private sector research institutions, funding agencies, trained personnel, pharmaceutical manufacturers, and equipment reside in the developed world, and are addressing developed country problems. Yet, the majority of the world's population and the greatest number of potentially preventable deaths occur in developing countries. Whereas the diseases of poverty due to infections, deficiencies, and hazards remain the major causes of death in the developing world (Preston, *et al.*, 1976), the diseases of affluence, such as cancer, cardiovascular, endocrine, and gastroenteric disorders, which are major killers in industrialized countries, are rising as well. Health research is generally accorded a low priority for national spending, and as a consequence, developing countries spend very little on research to solve their unique health problems.

It is clear in light of the above constraints that the process of assessing and setting priorities is an important facet of the management and implementation of health programs and research. This monograph presents a process for establishing such priorities. Setting priorities does not necessarily imply exclusivity. Other procedures may identify different priorities; and variations in societal, political, economic, and epidemiologic conditions will modify the outcome of the decision-making process. Above all, the setting of priorities involves consideration of the complex interactions between health and many other sectors in the society or community. Programs affecting health, for example, may have far-reaching implications in other spheres. The dilemma of evaluating alternatives is not easily tractable; however, use of the analytic framework presented here should help improve the efficient use of the limited available resources.

The priorities for program implementation may differ from the those for research. For example, with program implementation for health improvement, the priorities rest in the provision of those equitable, population-based interventions of proven efficacy that are inexpensive, cost-effective, technically feasible, and supported by the community, while concentrated on those most in need and the underserved. In contrast, *biomedical* research addresses those conditions for which no inexpensive, efficacious, technically feasible control measures yet exist, and these research priorities entail the development of better preventive or treatment methods. Other areas of research include *engineering improvements, epidemiology, operations and management, health systems evaluation, financing schemes,* and *methods for policy-making.*

The process for prioritizing research and program implementation commences with an analysis of the causes of morbidity and mortality in the developing world. Temporal trends and regional differences are considered. Processes for analyzing the health situation on a local, regional, or district level are presented. An evaluation of the interventions available for preventing or treating these causes of ill health is discussed with an analysis of efficacy and costs. To set priorities for biomedical research and development, those major causes of ill health that lack adequate interventions (*i.e.*, treatment or prevention is inefficacious, costly, or inconvenient for full compliance) must be identified. Prioritizing other types of research, such as epidemiology, health systems analysis, policy-making, and intersectoral analysis, entails an evaluation of the potential of each of these disciplines or methods to ultimately improve health. Any priorities identified must be modified in light of the costs of the research; the capability and location of the research institution; the likelihood of successful outcome; funding availability; flexibility; plurality; and other factors.

Setting priorities for implementation at the local level involves identification of burden of illness; available interventions and their cost-effectiveness; the feasibility, ease of implementation, and likelihood of success; and other factors.

This publication details the above outlined process and presents the available information with which organizations, such as multilateral and bilateral agencies, and governments, may prioritize health investments. For national, regional, or local policy and program decisions, a parallel process can take place in situations in which promoting health by minimizing deaths and disabling conditions remains the goal. Another process used for evaluating priorities for primary health care implementation involves broad-based review of the functioning of a particular health system nationwide, as set forth by the World Health Organization (WHO, 1982).

It is unfortunate that much of the information required for informed decision-making is simply not available. The author has reported the known information on global mortality and efficacy of interventions, as well as the few studies on cost-effectiveness found from literature survey. Several of the parameters, such as likelihood of success or significant breakthrough, cost of research or health service delivery programs, and present capacity, are not so well understood or vary enormously from place to place. Nevertheless, estimates can usually be made within a reasonable range of values and checked through discussion with scientists, public health officials in the developing world, administrators, and agency officials. Such a strictly quantitative evaluation, along with sensitivity analysis and testing of the robustness of the conclusions, was used for setting priorities for vaccine research by the Institute of Medicine (IOM, 1984 and 1986).

In many instances, rather than attempting to exactly quantify each parameter and then test (through sensitivity analyis) each type of health promotion program and health research option, the final conclusion rests upon qualitative opinion and consensus with other experts in the field. A more strictly quantitative comparison may be possible, however, using some of the recently developed decision-analysis computer programs.

Health Status (Burden of Illness)

Historical Trends

In the last 25 years, in practically all countries of the world, infant mortality rates have declined while life expectancy rates have increased. In 1983, fewer than ten countries had infant mortality rates greater than 150/1000 live births and none reported rates greater than 200/1000 (World Bank, 1987a). Post-neonatal infant mortality has decreased at a much faster rate than neonatal mortality. Childhood mortality rates have declined in a similar manner but are less well documented.

The causes of this health improvement are not entirely known. Improved socio-economic conditions have undoubtedly played some role. Education, particularly of women, and provision of health services and immunizations have also contributed (Halstead, *et al.*, 1985).

As immunizable and infectious diseases have declined in recent years, injuries have increased, becoming the second most important cause of infant, childhood, youth, and young adult morbidity and mortality. Figure 1 (p. 23) presents the overall experience of morbidity and mortality in Chilean children (Toucher, 1981). As shown, childhood injuries usually occur around the home, while injuries in youths and adults are more often the result of motor vehicle accidents, occupational injuries, and violence (Baker, 1984; Guyer, 1985; Hatton, 1986; Manciaux, 1986; Romer, 1986; Taket, 1986; Tursz, 1986; Wintmute, 1986). The incidence of motor vehicle and industrial injuries has increased precipitously in the developing world in conjunction with the proliferation of cars, trucks, roads, and factories. The larger factories are usually targeted in such statistical compilations, as they are the better monitored workplaces, but cottage industries and village workplaces are frequently more dangerous, since little effort may be made to ensure safety (Manciaux and Romer, 1986).

Another underlying cause of disease and death steadily rising in the third world is tobacco use, both smoking and smokeless (as in snuff or chewing tobacco). Anti-smoking campaigns have been given low priority, partly because of lack of realization of the health risks and partly because of the important economic status of the tobacco industry. Chronic obstructive pulmonary disease, lung cancer, and vascular disease secondary to smoking remain relatively minor public health problems in the poorest countries, but the accelerating incidence rates of disease and tobacco use foreshadow an epidemic beginning within the next decade.

In the last decade, a new infectious disease, the Acquired Immune Deficiency Syndrome (AIDS) caused by the Human Immunodeficiency Virus (HIV), was recognized first in the United States, then in Haiti and European nations, and finally world-wide. At present, the amount of disease and death remain small compared to other major public health problems, but AIDS, particularly in industrialized countries, may eventually overtax the health system because of the prolonged, expensive, skilled care needed to keep its victims alive. The extent of the epidemic is unknown. In this report, little will be said about AIDS, since an enormous research effort has already been mounted throughout the world funded by the USA and Western European countries (Quinn, *et al.*, 1986; Von Reyn and Mann, 1987). In addition, the AIDS Special Programme of the World Health Organization (WHO) is spearheading worldwide efforts and coordinating donor consensus for education, prevention, and treatment. The 1987 funding levels total almost $40 million, and the Programme estimates the budget will increase to over $600 million by the early 1990's. This figure does not include the cost of treatment, hospitalization, long-term care, or vaccine and drug development. Several bilateral agencies have coordinated activities with the WHO Programme. For example, the United States Agency for International Development (USAID) has committed more than $50 million to five-year projects which provide technical and program support for AIDS programs and assist in mounting extensive health education campaigns in developing countries, particularly Africa.

Present Global Status

Global mortality attributable to the major causes of death in 1980 in the different regions of the world and in the developed and developing areas is presented in Table 1 (Hakulinen, *et al.,* 1986). Table 2 presents estimates for the global prevalence (or incidence for short-term conditions) of death and number of episodes for the major morbid conditions of the developing world in 1986, ranked according to the number of deaths caused. The infectious diseases are disaggregated because, through the use of vaccines and chemotherapy, these are the most easily prevented and treated illnesses. The estimates are derived from the WHO, supplemented by published studies. The sources are given in the following discussions of the most prevalent diseases.

Since the major goal of public health is the prevention of premature mortality, a more powerful indicator of the relative importance of each of these conditions in causing premature death would be the calculation of years of potential life lost before the age of 65 attributable to each condition (Anonymous, 1986). Inadequate information on causes of death, age at onset, length of disability, and age at death for each of these diseases, however, makes it impossible to propose plausible estimations. The reader should bear in mind that these conditions affect very different age groups and thereby produce vastly different societal and familial burdens. Injuries, hepatitis-B-related hepatocellular carcinoma, and maternal mortality primarily affect young adults in the socio-economically active age group, and loss of a parent seriously affects the health of her or his children. Low birth weight, malaria, and diarrheal disease deaths occur largely among infants and children. The majority of deaths from diseases of the circulatory system and neoplasms take place among adults and the elderly.

Table 2 ranks these conditions by number of deaths caused, but this rating method tends to minimize the importance of those conditions which induce prolonged disability. Enormous societal costs result from diseases, such as leprosy and poliomyelitis—diseases which maim rather than kill.

The estimates derive from WHO studies and expansions of relatively small epidemiologic studies performed in various parts of the world. Table 2 is not based on communicable disease notifications, since case reporting is rarely complete even in highly developed countries and is often irregular in developing countries. The

Table 1. Annual death rates (/1000) due to major causes of death by age group and level of development, around 1980.

AGE GROUP (years)	LEVEL OF DEVELOP.	ALL CAUSES	INFECTIONS	NEO-PLASMS	CIRCULATORY SYSTEM	PREGNANCY	PERINATAL	INJURY	OTHER
0-14	World Total	12.0	6.4	0.1	0.3	0.00	2.1	0.4	2.8
	M*	2.1	0.5	0.1	0.1	0.00	0.7	0.2	0.6
	L	13.9	7.5	0.1	0.3	0.00	2.3	0.4	3.3
	LS	23.4	13.3	0.0	0.5	0.00	3.5	0.5	5.5
15-44	World Total	3.2	1.3	0.2	0.5	0.12		0.6	0.5
	M	1.4	0.1	0.2	0.3	0.01		0.6	0.2
	L	3.8	1.7	0.2	0.5	0.15		0.6	0.6
	LS	5.5	2.8	0.2	0.7	0.23		0.7	0.9
45-64	World Total	13.9	3.2	2.5	5.1	0.01		0.8	2.3
	M	8.5	0.4	2.7	4.1	0.00		0.6	0.7
	L	16.9	4.8	2.4	5.7	0.02		0.9	3.1
	LS	17.8	5.3	2.3	5.9	0.02		0.9	3.4
65 +	World Total	65.0	8.3	8.4	33.9			1.6	12.9
	M	57.0	4.0	9.9	35.3			1.5	6.3
	L	73.2	12.7	6.8	32.5			1.6	19.6
	LS	77.7	14.7	7.4	32.3			1.6	21.8

M is Developed Areas; L is Developing Areas; LS is Least Developed Areas. Source: Hakulinen et al., 1986.

Table 2. Causes of Death for Individuals of all Ages in the Developing World.

CONDITIONS	INFECTIONS[1]	DEATHS[1]	EPISODES[1]
Respiratory Disease (upper and lower)	—	10,000[2]	15,000,000[3]
Circulatory System[4]	—	8,000	*
(Low Birth Weight[5])	—	(5,000)	(19,000)
Diarrhea	—	4,300	2,8000,000
Measles[6]	67,000	2,000	67,000
Injuries	—	2,000	*
(Malnutrition[8])	—	(2,000)	(5-8,000)
Neoplasms[9]	—	2,000	*
Malaria	2,600,000[10]	1,500	150,000
P. falciparum	—	1,350	120,000
Tetanus	—	1,200	1,800
Tuberculosis	1,000,000	900	7,000
Hepatitis B[11]	300,000	800	3,700
Whooping Cough	55,000	600	51,000
Typhoid	70,000	600	35,000
Maternal Mortality	—	500	—
Meningitis	—	350	1,000,000
Schistosomiasis	200,000	250-500	10,000
Syphilis[12]	15,000	200	250
Amebiasis	500,000	70	40,000
Human Immunodeficiency Virus (HIV)	4,000	50-70	140
South American Trypanosomiasis	24,000	60	1,200
Rheumatic Fever and Heart Disease	—	52	2,200
Hookworm	800,000	50	1,500
Rabies	35	35	35
Diphtheria	60,000	30	600
Dengue	*	15	48
Hepatitis A	*	14	5,000
Yellow Fever	*	9	82
Japanese B Encephalitis	*	7	28
Ascariasis	700,000	<10	700
Giardiasis	250,000	<10	500
Poliomyelitis	150,000	2	220[13]
Leprosy	1,000	1	1,000
Leishmaniasis	1,000	1	1,000
Trichuriasis	500,000	<1	100
Filariasis	90,000	<1	1,000
Dracunculiasis	1,000	<1	1,000
Onchocerciasis[14]	1-5,000	<1	*
African Trypanosomiasis	*	<1	*
Other[15]	*	1-2,000	*

See next page for footnotes.

Table 2 Footnotes

1. (Thousands/yr.) Episodes means yearly occurrence of disease.

2. 4 million of these deaths occur in children under 5 years old.

3. 25 million episodes of acute lower respiratory tract infectious disease and 15 billion episodes of acute upper respiratory tract infectious disease.

4. This category includes cardiovascular diseases and certain degenerative diseases (nephritis, cirrhosis of the liver, ulcers of stomach and duodenum, and diabetes).

5. Low birth weight is the underlying cause of death, although the immediate cause may be respiratory, diarrheal or other disease; therefore, these deaths have also been counted in the other categories.

6. A small proportion of these deaths may also be counted in the diarrheal disease category.

7. Occurrences of injury are probably one hundred times more frequent than deaths, but extremely little reliable data are available on incidence.

8. Severe malnutrition is the underlying cause of death, although the immediate cause may be respiratory, diarrheal, or other disease; therefore, these deaths have also been counted in other categories.

9. Includes neoplasms of all types except Hepatitis B-related hepatocellular carcinoma which is listed separately.

10. This is the population at risk inhabiting infected areas; 365,000,000 live in highly endemic areas.

11. The infections are the asymptomatic carriers of hepatitis B surface antigen present in the world. Episodes include acute hepatitis, cirrhosis, and primary hepatocellular carcinoma.

12. The deaths are primarily excess perinatal deaths among the 10% of seroreactive women giving birth in sub-Saharan Africa. No good information is available on adult deaths from tertiary syphilis or extent of disease in other parts of the world.

13. Cases of paralysis.

14. No systematic survey of prevalence and incidence has occurred since the beginning of the onchocerciasis control program in West Africa, which has markedly diminished the occurrence of infection and disease.

15. Other. Deaths of unclear etiology or diseases with relatively small numbers of cases.

—   Not applicable

*   No data

efforts of the EPI, UNICEF, and other national and international agencies within the last few years to provide universal immunization have vastly improved the surveillance, monitoring, and reporting system for the immunization-preventable illnesses.

The bibliography lists the references upon which the estimates in Table 2 are based.

The problems with many of the global estimates include the generalizability of the small studies, which may only represent a peculiar ecological or epidemiologic niche, and double counting of illness and deaths, such as the childhood deaths that result from an accumulation of health insults (malnutrition, low birth weight, measles, and diarrhea). The question arises, should a death under these circumstances be attributed to measles, diarrhea, malnutrition, or low birth weight, since preventing any one of these illnesses may not have averted the death.

Of all the illnesses listed in Table 2, infectious diseases are the most easily prevented and cured given the available technology. Control of these diseases is responsible for the enormous increases in life expectancy occurring in the developed countries in the last century. Improved socio-economic conditions, nutritional status, education, and health services have also contributed to the decline in morbidity and mortality. For example, in England, in 1881, when life expectancy at birth was only 47 years, the probability of eventually dying from an infectious disease was above 40%, while in 1964, when life expectancy at birth was 70 + years, the probability was only 13% of dying from infection (Preston, 1976).

It is clear that the developing world is amidst a transition, which results in suffering not only from the diseases of poverty (excessive burden of infectious and tropical disease, hazards, and deficiencies), but also from a rising prevalence of the diseases of affluence common to the developed world. Infectious diseases are the most easily controlled. Yet even though they may be decreasing in some areas, they remain the major cause of illness.

Major Diseases of the Developing World—Description and Status

The major disorders causing death and illness in the developing world are described below with regard to epidemiology, importance, and currently available interventions. The conditions are presented in descending order in terms of the number of deaths each produces annually. The estimates are based on the 1986 population distribution.

- *Respiratory Disease.*   This entity heads the list as the major infectious cause of death. Inclusive of diarrheal disease, it is responsible for half to two thirds of the morbidity and mortality from communicable diseases in the developing world (Berman and McIntosh, 1986; WHO, 1986b). Many different organisms can cause respiratory infections and each requires a different drug for treatment and unique vaccine for prevention. Table 3 lists the more common pathogens. A large proportion of the cases do not identify the causative pathogen, probably because present diagnostic techniques are so difficult to perform in the field. Unlike diarrheal disease, which can be treated with oral rehydration and largely prevented with handwashing and appropriate use of water and sanitation, there is no tested, simple control measure for respiratory diseases. Each pathogen requires an ideal antibiotic or antiviral agent for treatment or prophylaxis, and each must have a separately formulated immunogen to produce immunity. Throughout the world, the incidence of acute upper respiratory tract infections appears to be the same: for those under 5 years it amounts to 5-6 episodes annually, decreasing to about 2 per year for adults. In developing countries, children suffer from lower respiratory complications several times more frequently than children in industrialized nations, and these children are therefore at much higher risk of death (Berman, *et al.,* 1983; Cochi, *et al.,* 1985; Davenport, 1982; Douglas and Kerby-Eaton, 1985; Glezen, *et al.,* 1982; Gwaltney, 1982; Kielmann, *et al.,* 1983; Lennette, 1981; Leowski, 1986; Monto, 1982; PAHO, 1983; Pio, *et al.,* 1985; Riley, 1985; Riley, *et al.,* 1986; Shann, *et al.,* 1985a,b; Stansfield, 1987; WHO, 1986b,c,d).

Table 3.   Primary Pathogens Causing Death From Acute Respiratory Infections Among Children Under 5 Years of Age.

ORGANISMS	PROPORTION OF DEATHS (%)
S. pneumoniae	22.5
H. influenzae	11.5
Influenza virus	10
Respiratory syncytial virus	7
Parainfluenza virus	5.5
Staphylococcus aureus	4.4
Others	39.1
Total	100%

Modified from: Institute of Medicine, 1986.

• *Diseases of the Circulatory System.* These include cardiovascular and certain degenerative diseases such as nephritis, cirrhosis of the liver, ulcers of the stomach and duodenum, and diabetes. They affect primarily adults and the elderly, and few control measures are available. Hypertension treatment, diet, smoking prevention, and exercise may have some influence on mortality rates, but require long-term behavioral modifications. The infectious causes of circulatory illness (Chagas disease and rheumatic heart disease) are listed separately; however, these represent a tiny percentage of episodes and deaths. More deaths in in this category will occur in the future as people live longer, their diet and exercise patterns change, and smoking increases (Hakulinen *et al.,* 1986).

• *Low Birth Weight.* This condition is assigned when the birth weight is 2500 grams or less. In many industrialized countries as few as 4% of all infants belong to this category at birth, but in some parts of the developing world almost 50% of babies begin life disadvantaged by low birth weight (Petros-Barvazian and Behar, 1978; Puffer and Serrano, 1987; Villar, *et al.,* 1986; WHO, 1984). The consequences of low birth weight are myriad. In developing countries, few of these infants achieve the normal weight-for-age by even 3 years, and the majority are malnourished with all its attendant problems (Paine, *et al.,* 1983). The risk of dying in infancy and childhood is many times that of a normal weight baby. For example, in a recent study from the USA, although low-birth-weight infants represented only 6% of live births, they comprised 55% of infant deaths (Ashworth and Feachem, 1985b; Puffer and Serrano, 1987). The risk of developmental disabilities and retardation in mental and motor skills in this group is also high (IOM, 1985).

Low birth weight results from either preterm delivery; that is, the fetus grows normally during pregnancy but the gestation is shorter than 37 weeks, or from slow intrauterine growth but normal gestational duration. A few severely affected infants suffer from both intrauterine growth retardation (IUGR) and short gestation. In industrialized countries, about two thirds of the low-birth-weight babies are preterm; but in developing countries, most appear to result from IUGR, although the data base is probably inadequate (Puffer and Serrano, 1987). Small improvements in the incidence of low birth weight will markedly decrease the infant and child mortality rate. For example, a fall in prevalence from 30% to 15% could result in a fall in the infant mortality rate of around 25%; *e.g.,* from 160/1000 to 120/1000 (Ashworth and Feachem, 1985b).

Few interventions are known to prevent prematurity: malaria chemoprophylaxis or control in areas hyperendemic for *P. falciparum*, nutritional supplementation throughout the pregnancy targeted to extremely malnourished mothers or women under conditions of severe food shortage and excess physical exertion, in addition to stopping smoking, will improve birth weights (Ashworth and Feachem, 1985b; IOM, 1985; Lechtig, *et al.*, 1978; McDonald, *et al.*, 1981; Mora, *et al.*, 1979; Prentice, *et al.*, 1985; Rush, *et al.*, 1980; Viegas, *et al.*, 1982). Otherwise, more research into the causes and possible preventive measures, particularly gestational infections precipitating early delivery or affecting intrauterine growth rates, is greatly needed. For example, maternal Group B streptococcus infection appears to cause both prematurity and maternal morbidity and mortality. Control of this infection by immunization or targeted treatment could prevent a substantial proportion of this burden (Walsh, in press). Prematurity is listed in parentheses in Table 2 because the infants and children affected by low birth weight usually die from respiratory infection or diarrheal disease, and these deaths are counted in these categories.

• *Diarrheal Disease.*   The next most common infectious cause of death in the developing world is diarrheal disease. A great variety of pathogens produce this syndrome, and Table 4 lists the more common organisms. In spite of the multiple etiologies, most cases can be treated and deaths averted through the use of oral rehydration (Feachem, *et al.*, 1982). Only those severe cases of bloody diarrhea and dysentery caused largely by ameba, Shigella, and enteropathogenic *E. coli.* will not respond to oral rehydration. In developing countries, adults usually suffer from at least one episode of mild diarrhea yearly. In contrast, children under 5 have an incidence of 2 to 10 episodes of diarrhea annually, averaging about 4 in most poor communities. This dehydrating illness lasts several days to a week (Rohde, 1986).

Malnutrition and diarrhea appear to interact with one another. Diarrhea contributes to malnutrition through a variety of mechanisms, including anorexia and intestinal malabsorption, while malnourished individuals are at increased risk of prolonged illness and death when stricken with diarrhea (Rohde, 1986). The use of oral rehydration solutions containing rice water or enriched with short-chain peptides seems to avert many of the nutritional deficits. The standard oral rehydration solution available in packets con-

Table 4. Primary Pathogens Causing Deaths From Diarrheal Disease.

ORGANISM	PROPORTION OF DEATHS (%)
Rotavirus	20
Enterotoxigenic *E. coli.*	18
Shigella	15
Cholera	3
Salmonella	1
Others (Amebiasis, giardia, campylobacter, aeromonas, cryptosporidium, etc.)	43
Total	100%

Modified from: Institute of Medicine, 1986.

tains only a small amount of calories from sugar, but the calorie-dense varieties provide nutritional support, while still treating the dehydration. Increasing food intake during the recovery period will also help prevent malnutrition (Ashworth and Feachem, 1985a,b,c; De Zoysa and Feachem, 1985a,b; Feachem, 1983; Feachem and Koblinsky, 1984).

Provision of adequate water supplies and sanitation decreases the incidence and mortality from diarrhea by approximately 20%. The joint UNDP/World Bank Water Decade Program, together with UNICEF and other agencies, has developed low-cost hand pumps and latrines, contributing to the widespread increase in the presence of these facilities world-wide. Presence, however, does not translate automatically into appropriate use. Installations must be accompanied by education and commitment to appropriate use and maintenance (Cvjetanovic, 1986; Clemens and Stanton, 1987; Esrey, *et al.*, 1985; Esrey and Habicht, 1986; Feachem, 1984; Feachem, *et al.*, 1982; Feachem and Koblinsky, 1983; Phillips, *et al.*, 1987).

• *Measles.* Essentially, everyone who is not immunized and who survives beyond the first six months of life eventually becomes infected with measles and suffers from the illness. Particularly the very young and the malnourished suffer severe and prolonged disease with multiple complications, including diarrhea, pneumonia, otitis media, and enormous weight loss that can lead to malnutrition (Walsh, 1986). Case fatality rates in community studies range from 1% to 10%; therefore, this preventable infection may cause more than 5% of *all* deaths and more than 20% of all infant and child deaths (Feachem and Koblinsky, 1983; Walsh, 1986). Particularly in cities, infants contract measles when they are less than one year old. Case fatality is highest in this age group. Unfortunately, the vaccine is ineffective for infants younger than nine months, but immunization of all infants nine months of age or older will largely eliminate this deadly disease. In the last decade, global immunization coverage has increased spectacularly, to the extent that now over 45% of infants and children have been immunized against measles (WHO, 1987). Social mobilization; nationwide campaigns; WHO, UNICEF, UNDP and other international agencies; private voluntary organizations; bilateral agencies; among other groups, have made universal childhood immunization a major priority. UNICEF and the WHO/Expanded Programme on Immunization (EPI) have spearheaded these remarkably successful efforts. The EPI price for the current vaccine is six cents a dose purchased through UNICEF suppliers (EPI, personal communication, 1987).

• *Injuries.*   Death rates from injuries are uncannily similar in all regions of the world, but few systems gather data about the frequency of their occurrence (Hakulinen, *et al.*, 1986). In the developing world, only a small proportion of the population has access to the sophisticated health services frequently needed to treat injuries. Thus, injuries probably result in death more often in developing countries than in industrialized regions.

Young adults and children have the greatest risk of injuries, usually as a result of exposure to hazardous and unsafe environments in the community, home, and at work. In Chile, following the widespread introduction and usage of childhood immunizations and oral rehydration, injuries have superceded respiratory diseases as the most common cause of childhood deaths (Figure 1) (Toucher, 1981). Injuries result most often from burns, motor vehicle accidents, and falls (Manciaux and Romer, 1986). The loss of these healthy, productive individuals incurs an inordinately great societal cost. Little is presently known about risk factors or the appropriate interventions to prevent these episodes, but a substantial proportion of these accidents are certainly preventable. In the United States, education and improved environmental safety appear to have effected a decline in the incidence of injuries in the last several decades. The potential exists for a substantial decline

Figure 1. Mortality in Chilean Children 1-4 Years

From: Diarrheal, Respiratory, and Vaccine-Preventable Diseases; and Accidents and Violence, in the Triennia 1962-1964, 1969-1971, and 1976-1978, for Both Sexes.[1]

per 100,000

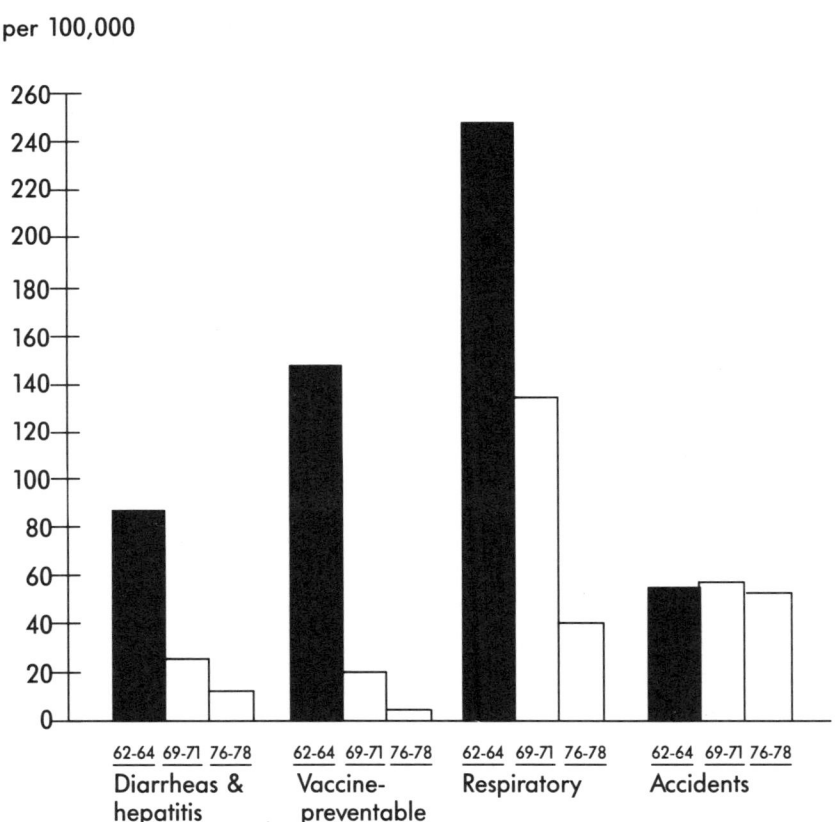

[1]Rates calculated by applying the proportions of the deaths due to these causes as published in the Demographic Annual of the National Institute of Statistics, to the rates obtained through the Greville method.

Source: Toucher, 1981.

in injury incidence and mortality world-wide. However, epidemiologic research to identify locally important risk factors and introduce appropriate interventions such as education, behavior change, and improved cooking stoves are prerequisite (Baker, 1984; Guyer and Gallagher, 1985; Hatton *et al.*, 1986; Manciaux and Romer, 1986; Taket, 1986; Tursz, 1986; Romer and Manciaux, 1986; Wintemute, 1986).

• *Malnutrition.* This can be defined as a state in which the physical function of an individual is impaired to the point where she or he can no longer maintain an adequate level of performance during physical work, in resisting or recovering from the effects of disease, in maintaining an adequate level of growth, or in sustaining the processes of pregnancy or lactation. This impairment does not result from any other known disease process. To avoid malnutrition, a family must be able to do physical work on their land and crops, or to sell their labor for cash. The returns must be sufficient not only to secure their immediate food needs, but also to sustain productivity over long periods, and to survive through bad years as well as good. They must, additionally, be able to adjust total production from their resources to keep pace with the number of dependents in the family. Malnourished individuals can no longer sustain their existence because of their physical disability.

Nutritional status must be considered both as the outcome of the process of acquiring, consuming, and utilizing food, and as one of the key inputs into that process. The food an individual eats determines the amount of effort he or she can use to secure food in the future. Figure 2 illustrates the factors influencing nutritional status (Payne, 1985).

The objective measurements for nutritional status include weight-for-age, skin-fold thickness, triceps circumference, weight-for-height, and height-for-age, which are compared to national or international standards. Nutritional surveys primarily include children. The estimate for morbidity and mortality in Table 2 refers to this age group.

Inequality of resources, poverty, and social discrimination remain the foremost causes of malnutrition. Changes in the system of food production and distribution, which leave these conditions unchanged, also leave malnutrition unchanged. Humans can adapt to a fairly wide range of dietary situations, but only when that adaptive capacity is stretched beyond its limits does the body fail to

Figure 2.   Factors Influencing Nutritional Status[1]

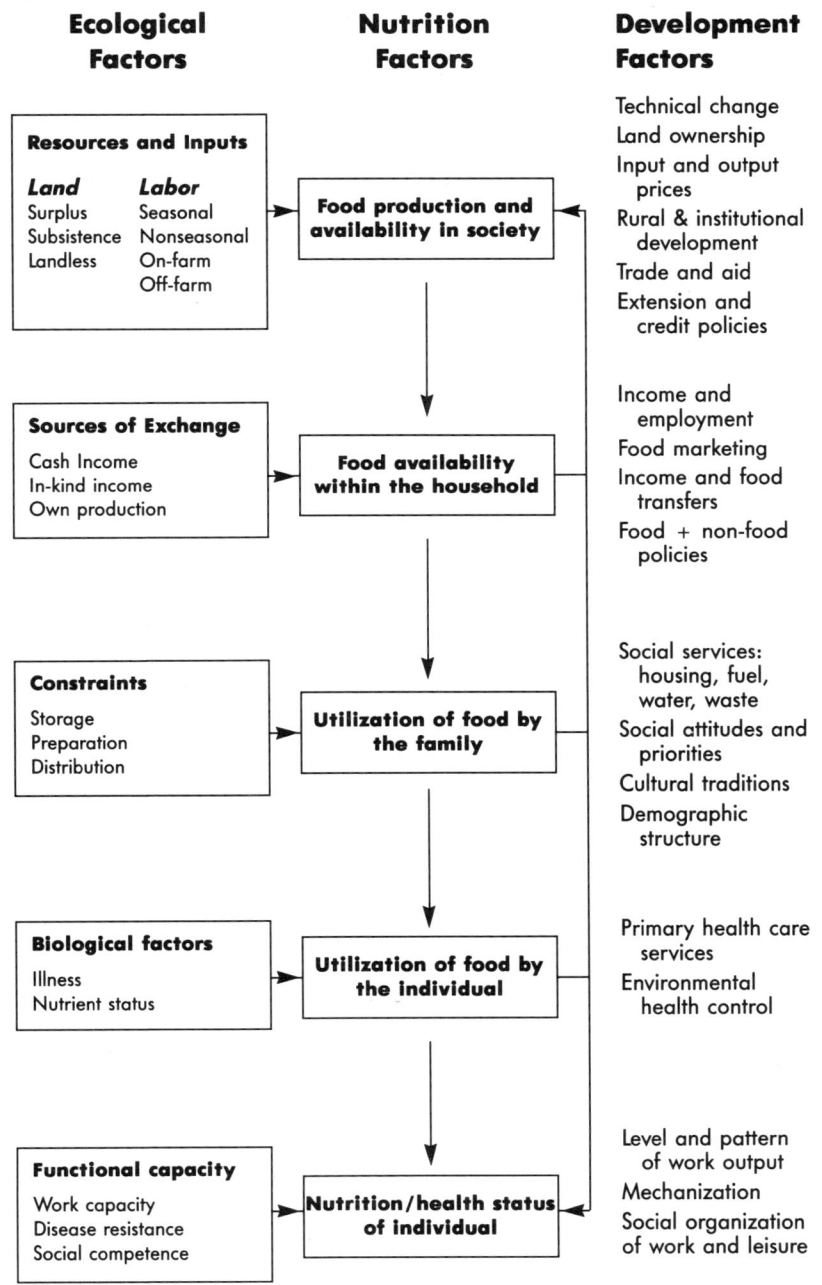

Ecological Factors	Nutrition Factors	Development Factors

Ecological Factors

Resources and Inputs

Land	**Labor**
Surplus	Seasonal
Subsistence	Nonseasonal
Landless	On-farm
	Off-farm

Sources of Exchange

Cash Income
In-kind income
Own production

Constraints

Storage
Preparation
Distribution

Biological factors

Illness
Nutrient status

Functional capacity

Work capacity
Disease resistance
Social competence

Nutrition Factors

Food production and availability in society

Food availability within the household

Utilization of food by the family

Utilization of food by the individual

Nutrition/health status of individual

Development Factors

Technical change
Land ownership
Input and output prices
Rural & institutional development
Trade and aid
Extension and credit policies

Income and employment
Food marketing
Income and food transfers
Food + non-food policies

Social services: housing, fuel, water, waste
Social attitudes and priorities
Cultural traditions
Demographic structure

Primary health care services
Environmental health control

Level and pattern of work output
Mechanization
Social organization of work and leisure

maintain its functional capacity, and malnutrition ensues. This means that the extent of real malnutrition, *i.e.*, physiological states carrying penalties in terms of loss of function as distinct from otherwise benign deviations of growth or body size, is much less frequent than previously believed, but such *real* malnutrition is concentrated amongst the most economically and socially deprived sections of the population.

Nutrition and infections are intimately related. Infections, particularly diarrhea, exert a negative impact on nutritional status, while malnutrition predisposes the individual to an increased risk of morbidity and mortality from various infections. In Bangladesh, the mortality rate of the children in the lowest 10%, according to weight-for-age or height-for-age, exceeds the rate of those in the top 10% by a factor of four (Chen, 1986; Chen, *et al.*, 1980). Epidemiological studies in Guatemala, the Gambia, and Bangladesh have demonstrated a marked negative relationship between infections and child physical growth and development (Mata, 1978; Mata, *et al.*, 1972; Martorell, *et al.*, 1975; Rowland, *et al.*, 1977). Diarrhea, measles, and malaria appear to have the greatest impact on nutrition (Keusch and Scrimshaw, 1986; Puffer and Serrano, 1973; Walsh, 1986). These diseases probably exert their effect through the mechanisms of decreased food intake, malabsorption, and loss of nutrients in the gastrointestinal tract during certain diarrheal diseases. Control of these infections should greatly lessen the burden of malnutrition in society. Enough food is produced in the world today to meet the physiological demands of all the individuals inhabiting this planet, if only equitably distributed. In spite of this, the number of malnourished children has changed but imperceptibly in the last few decades (Biswas and Pinstrup-Andersen, 1986).

Figure 2 gives an oversimplified view of the complex relationships and processes involved in nutrition (Payne, 1985). Note that the nutritional status of the individual is represented both as a "state" and as an "input" to the food production process. Hence, nutritional status measures the performance of the whole system.

How can malnutrition be treated or averted? Many of the more conventional types of nutrition programs have had disappointing results—promoting the production of specially nutritious foods, special food delivery systems aimed at young children, projects to educate people about the nutritional value of foods (Beaton and Ghassemi, 1982; Payne, 1985). Further attempts are needed to identify more effective alternatives to improve conventional programs.

The policy implications of malnutrition involve distinguishing a number of components of the problem (Joy, 1980). Table 5 outlines this approach. The most important distinctions are: (1) the existence of people currently suffering from malnutrition and needing treatment, (2) the enumeration and description of those categories of households at greatest risk of malnutrition either continuously or periodically, and (3) the processes (including infectious diseases) contributing to the increase or decrease of the numbers of families in those high-risk situations. Programs can be directed at any or all of these levels: identification and treatment or rehabilitation of those currently malnourished, monitoring the high-risk groups to avert deterioration of present status, control of infectious disease, and attempts to influence those processes augmenting malnutrition.

- *Neoplasms.* This category includes all the benign and malignant neoplasms affecting humankind (Hakulinen, *et al.,* 1986). Only a few of the less common types, such as childhood leukemia and Hodgkin's disease, can occasionally be cured. However, one of the most common types in the developing world, hepatitis-B-related hepatocellular carcinoma (listed separately in Table 2 p. 15), can now be prevented through the immunization of newborns. Adults and the elderly are the age groups most commonly affected by cancers. Lung cancer is rapidly increasing in incidence in the developing world following the epidemic increase in the use of tobacco (Muller, 1978). Years of research absorbing more than one billion dollars annually have not yet resulted in cures or preventions for the most common types of cancer, and prospects for rapid advances remain dim.

- *Malaria.* Particularly in sub-Saharan Africa, malaria causes an enormous number of deaths (Bruce-Chwatt, 1980; IOM, 1986; Malaria Action Programme, 1986; Parasitic Diseases Programme, 1986). Disaggregating malarial morbidity from other diseases is a difficult task because most people living in endemic areas who are infected remain totally asymptomatic. Several studies have demonstrated mortality declines of nearly one third in infants and adults as a result of insecticide spraying. These results probably are a better indication of the true burden of illness from this protozoan (Kuznetsov, 1977; Payne, *et al.,* 1976). The epidemiologic

Table 5.   Policy Issues of Malnutrition

PROBLEM:	TASK:
1. The existence of people currently malnourished.	The identification and treatment of the malnourished.
2. The existence of people in situations that are characterized by an unacceptable risk of malnutrition.	The reduction of the number of people exposed chronically to the risk of malnutrition.
3. Trends and forces that increase the numbers at risk of malnutrition.	Reducing or offsetting those forces which make for increase in the numbers at risk of malnutrition.
4. Lack of sensitivity and/or effective response by society to the above realities.	Improving sensitivity and responsiveness of society to nutritional deprivation.

studies evaluating field sites for future testing of malarial vaccine and the vaccine trials, themselves, will probably provide the most valid means of measuring the malaria burden of illness. The current control methods include: (1) attack on the parasite in the human host through the use of antimalarial drugs either for treatment of disease or for prophylaxis to prevent illness; (2) development of malarial vaccines; however, an effective vaccine will probably not be available for at least another decade; (3) reduction of contact between humans and mosquitoes through the use of screening, bed nets, and repellents; (4) reduction of mosquito breeding sites by environmental alterations, such as filling or draining collections of water, straightening and clearing streams and rivers, and intermittently drying irrigated fields; (5) attack on the larval stages of the mosquito through chemical and biologic interventions; (6) destruction of the adult mosquito by environmental or household spraying with pesticides (Bradley, *et al.*, 1986; Miller, *et al.*, 1986; Reubush, *et al.*, 1986). In light of the extensive spread of protozoal resistance to antimalarials and the pesticide resistance found among many mosquito species, source reduction through the use of environmental modification is becoming a more valuable malaria prevention scheme (PEEM, 1986).

• *Tetanus.* About two thirds of the deaths from tetanus occur in the neonatal period as a result of contamination of the umbilical stump with *Clostridium tetani.* The organism is commonly present in the environment, and thus minor soilage can result in infection. Neonatal tetanus can be prevented by immunizing pregnant women against tetanus and/or by training birth attendants in the use of clean techniques for delivery, especially sterile tools for cutting the cord. Non-neonatal tetanus occurs as a result of dirty wounds and can be prevented by administering tetanus immunization to children followed by booster doses about every ten years. The underlying cause of these deaths is injuries; adding these non-neonatal tetanus deaths to the injury category increases the evidence for the enormity of the societal burden from injuries (Arnold, *et al.*, 1986; Ross, 1986).

• *Tuberculosis.* Despite decades of BCG (Bacillus Calmette-Guerain) immunization and drug treatment, the incidence of new cases and deaths from tuberculosis (TB) essentially has not changed. The efficacy of BCG remains questionable even though it is the mainstay of TB control in many countries. Cure requires multiple drugs and many months of compliance, an extremely difficult task. Practically all adults in developing countries have been infected as indicated by skin test reactivity, but fewer than 5% develop clinical disease. Several of the risk factors for the development of clinical disease include age when first exposed, intensity of exposure, presence of other significant illnesses, pregnancy, and recent exposure. These factors, however, explain only a small proportion of the clinical cases. TB is a disease of young adults, the age group most economically active and productive in society, and of the impoverished. The challenge for current control programs is to increase and maintain compliance given the current lengthy course of drugs required for cure. The challenge for biomedical research is the discovery of a better, more efficacious immunization and a successful short-term drug treatment (Bulla, 1977; Clemens, *et al.*, 1983; Daniel, 1986; EPI, 1986; Guan-Quing, 1987; Pamra, 1987; Shapiro, *et al.*, 1985; WHO, 1986e).

• *Hepatitis B Virus.*   Among the diseases related to hepatitis B virus, hepatocellular carcinoma and cirrhosis of the liver carry the greatest disability and highest mortality rates (Beasley, *et al.*, 1981; Francis, 1986; Szmuness, *et al.*,1982). These sequelae begin to appear in young adulthood and the incidence peaks between 35 and 40 years of age, at least 20 years following initial exposure to the virus and onset of chronic infection. At present several long-term studies on the efficacy of the vaccine in preventing acquisition of chronic carriage of the virus and in ultimately preventing the mortal consequences of hepatoma and cirrhosis are under way in West Africa and East Asia. Results will not be known for at least 20 years. The vaccine has been quite expensive compared to the childhood immunizations ($100 + per dose compared to a few cents). But the new recombinant form, synthesized in yeast cells containing the gene for the hepatitis surface antigen (the first vaccine manufactured using the new powerful biomedical techniques), should reduce costs. The Korean plasma-derived vaccine costs only $1.00 per dose.

• *Whooping Cough (Pertussis).*   Like measles, this disease is highly contagious and affects essentially all children who do not obtain at least two doses of the immunization. Three doses have induced immunity in over 80% of children for many years, and the disease in non-immune adults is generally mild. The case fatality rate from pertussis and secondary complications is approximately 1%. The prolonged spasmodic cough during the illness frequently interferes with adequate nutritional intake and predisposes to malnutrition. The adverse effects of the vaccine have been greatly exaggerated, particularly when compared with the severity of the illness. Immunization acceptance has accelerated in the last several years largely due to social mobilization. UNICEF and the WHO Expanded Programme on Immunization (EPI) have led a global campaign which has gained widespread support among multilateral and bilateral agencies, heads of state and national governments, and private organizations. The three doses of the vaccine itself cost pennies. Particularly when combined with other vaccines, immunization programs become remarkably effective in terms of cost per death averted (EPI, 1985; Hewlitt, 1986; WHO, 1987).

- *Typhoid.* Approximately 75% of cases of this disease occur among school children and young adults (IOM, 1986). The currently available immunization for typhoid gives good protection but has never been universally administered because (1) it induces side effects in a large proportion of recipients, (2) confidence in its efficacy has been poor, and (3) the short duration of immunity necessitates boosters every 3 to 4 years to ensure maintenance of immunity. Several newer vaccines are presently undergoing large-scale clinical trials, but the results of these studies have generally been disappointing (IOM, 1986; Germanier and Furer, 1975). Even following the most optimistic schedule, these new vaccines will probably not be available for at least 5 to 7 years. Typhoid transmission occurs most commonly by contamination of food by intestinal carriers of the organism (Feachem, *et al.,* 1983). Provision of adequate water supplies, effective sanitary disposal, and personal hygiene should produce a substantial drop in incidence rates because of the interruption of spread from carriers to susceptibles. In many endemic areas, such as Lesotho and the South African black townships, provision of chlorinated water had no effect on the incidence of disease (Feachem, *et al.,* 1977). Provision of an adequate quantity of water is prerequisite, however, for careful personal hygiene. Cleaning of hands prior to handling food is key for the prevention of this disease, and *adequate quantity* of water available in the household rather than pristine quality *appears imperative.*

- *Maternal Mortality.* The public health community has only recently recognized the enormity of maternal mortality and its far-reaching consequences for family health. Efforts to define the most efficacious and cost-effective preventive measures are just beginning. According to WHO estimates, about 500,000 women die annually as a result of pregnancy. When a mother dies, usually her newborn dies too; and any other living children lose their primary caregiver and are placed at great risk. The primary causes of mortality during pregnancy are hemorrhage, severe infection (sepsis), toxemia (or eclampsia), and obstructed labor (Editorial, 1987). Several studies demonstrated that one third or more of these deaths occurs quite early in pregnancy as a result of primitive abortion attempts to terminate unwanted pregnancies (Herz and Measham, 1987). These deaths could be easily prevented by provision of family planning information and services to all women. These services would also promote the woman's ability to time and space her pregnancies to ensure good health at the time pregnancy begins. The World Bank estimates that up to 45% of maternal mortality may be averted through the provision and widespread use of family planning (Herz and Measham, 1987). Identifying the most appropriate and cost-effective methods for ensuring prenatal and delivery care for those at greatest risk awaits further research. Programs can then be modified to fit into the social, cultural, economic, and environmental constraints of local areas. At this point, however, the commonly used indicators of high risk are both insensitive and nonspecific. Although application of such indicators in most developing countries identifies 50% or more of all women as high risk, only half of the complications may occur among the high-risk group (Rinehart, *et al.*, 1984; WHO, 1985).

- *Meningitis.* Like diarrhea and respiratory infections, many different organisms can cause meningitis, and infants and children comprise the age group that most frequently suffers from this disease. The most common invading organisms are listed in Table 6. Two of the most common organisms, *Streptococcus pneumoniae* and *H. influenza B*, are also among the most common respiratory pathogens. Each of these different microorganisms requires a different vaccine for prevention, and in fact, vaccines for two of them contain antigens from numerous different strains (pneumococcus contains 23 antigens and meningococcus at least four).

Table 6.   Primary Pathogens Causing Deaths From Meningitis

ORGANISM	PROPORTION OF DEATHS (%)
S. pneumoniae	59
H. influenza B	28
N. meningitidis	10
Others	3
Total	100%

Modified from: Institue of Medicine, 1986.

Those who survive an episode of meningitis have a high risk of subsequent neurological and developmental problems. Currently, antibiotics are available for treatment when an episode occurs, but the patient must have ready access to health services in order to begin treatment promptly. One-dose schedules are used in epidemic situations in which those affected can only be reached by mobile teams or the extent of illness overwhelms the health system (Greenwood, 1986).

• *Schistosomiasis.*   Illness from schistosomiasis primarily affects school children and young adults. Drugs that treat, prevent, and decrease transmission of this disease are available, although they remain too expensive to be administered universally. This helminth infection has increased in several areas of the world, ironically spread through water and irrigation schemes planned to benefit agriculture and animal husbandry. Current strategies for the control of schistome infection, with its associated morbidity and mortality, include: (1) reduction of adult worm burdens, and hence of egg excretion, by chemotherapy; (2) reduction of environmental contamination, by health education and improved sanitation; (3) reduction in the numbers of intermediate hosts, by the use of molluscicides and the modification of habitats; and (4) reduction of exposure to infection following the installation of clean water supplies, and health education. Protected water and sanitary excreta disposal definitely inhibit transmission; however, chemotherapy given to at-risk populations appears to be the most cost-effective control measure currently available (Doumenge and Mott, 1984; Parasitic Diseases Programme, 1986; Warren, 1986).

- *Sexually Transmitted Diseases.*   Particularly in sub-Saharan Africa, the high prevalence of sexually transmitted diseases such as syphilis, gonorrhoea, and Acquired Immune Deficiency Syndrome (AIDS), has only recently been recognized. Infertility resulting from gonorrhoea and chlamydia affects up to 30% of women in some areas, particularly in Gabon, Uganda, Zaire, and the Central African Republic (Cates, *et al.*, 1985; Frank, 1983; Mabey, *et al.*, 1985; Meheus, *et al.*, 1980; Meheus, *et al.*, 1986). An average of 10% of pregnant women in several countries of Africa are serologically positive for syphilis (CDC, 1986; Friedmann and Wright, 1977; Hira, 1982a,b). Infection with the human immunodeficiency virus (HIV) which causes AIDS has been detected in 100 countries and in some areas affects up to 5% of the population (see below). The rapid social, cultural, and economic changes, particularly the spectacular increases in urban populations living in squatter settlements, the cyclic famines, and wars displacing people from their traditional homes and families, have likely contributed to an increase in family separation, promiscuity, and transmission of venereal diseases.

The consequences of untreated syphilis in pregnancy are formidable. For example, a careful study from the 1940's prior to the widespread use of penicillin demonstrated that a stillbirth results in approximately 20% of pregnancies, syphilitic infants in about one third, and neonatal deaths in about 12% (CDC, 1986; Friedmann and Wright, 1977; Ratnam, *et al.*, 1980 and 1982). Repeating such a study comparing treated and untreated women would, of course, be unethical now. Seroreactive pregnant women are about five times more likely to have a spontaneous abortion or stillbirth compared with uninfected women (CDC, 1986). Syphilitic infants have neurological and anatomical congenital defects and frequently grow poorly both in utero and postnatally. Their risk of developing severe complications from other diseases is therefore excessive (Larsson and Larsson, 1970). Detection and treatment with one dose of long-acting penicillin can prevent pregnancy losses, developmental consequences, and the late complications of syphilis in the mother, but such a program is not easily administered. First, it requires recognition of the magnitude of the problem. Second, an institution must be identified for diagnostic and treatment services. Third, research must be conducted to identify the most cost-effective methods of providing these services. Encouraging use of condoms, health education, follow-up, and treatment of contacts will help control the spread of these diseases.

• *Amebiasis.* Among parasitic infections, only malaria and schistosomiasis exceed these protozoa in killing more individuals annually (Walsh, 1985). Even though this intestinal infection can cause diarrhea, oral rehydration usually does not help, since the diarrhea associated with amebiasis is not watery, but contains blood and mucus. Drug therapy for as little as three days will cure most individuals with the intestinal dysentery or hepatic abscess (Guarner, 1986). Provision of adequate water supplies and sanitation have had mixed effects on the prevalence of infection, but this finding is probably related to the infrequent use of these facilities and poor personal hygiene of the users (Walsh and Martinez-Palomo, 1986). Treatment of food handlers who carry the organism asymptomatically and improvement of personal hygiene will probably have the greatest impact on decreasing the prevalence of amebiasis, although in the long run, water and sanitation must be improved world-wide.

• *Human Immunodeficiency Virus (HIV) and Acquired Immune Deficiency Syndrome (AIDS).* From the first recognition of cases of this disease in 1979, AIDS has rapidly increased in incidence and scope to its present form as a global health problem. At least 100 countries have reported cases, with more than 44,000 cases in the United States, nearly 3,000 cases in Europe, and many thousands suspected in Africa (Von Reyn and Mann, 1987). WHO estimates that at least 1.5 million people world-wide have been infected with the causative agent called human immunodeficiency virus (HIV); however, several types of the virus have been recognized and these may vary in their potential for eventually producing AIDS. The majority of those affected are young adults in the economically and socially most productive years of life. An increasing number of children are infected from their mothers or possibly through other agents, such as reuse of non-sterilized needles. Within 5 years following infection with the virus, between 10% and 30% develop clinical disease (Quinn, *et al.,* 1986; Von Reyn and Mann, 1987), but the long-term consequences of infection are not well known. Each year, investigators identify more illnesses that result from infection with the virus; for example, thrombocytopenia, cancers of various types, and neurological deterioration and dementia. Unfortunately, those infected who do not develop AIDS seem likely to develop other sicknesses many years following infection. In the industrialized nations, care for AIDS patients during the prolonged disease threatens to overwhelm the capacity of health care institutions and bankrupt the system. In Africa and South America, the disease is rapidly increasing in importance although the classical bacterial, viral, and parasitic illnesses continue to cause many times more deaths and episodes of disability.

Present treatments produce only temporary remission and do not cure. A huge proportion of the biomedical research capacity in the United States and Europe is now devoted to analyzing this virus and disease and to discovering means for cure and prevention. A prototype vaccine has begun human trials, but testing and licensing will probably require five to ten years. Present control measures are limited to: educational efforts to change the behaviors associated with transmission, treatment of the intercurrent infections resulting from the immunosuppression caused by the disease, and antiviral treatment. Several different patterns of transmission occur; however, the reason transmission varies is still unclear. In industrialized countries, multiple homosexual partners, intravenous drug use, needle sharing, and transfusion with blood products carry the greatest risk, while in developing countries, having multiple *heterosexual* partners carries the greatest risk. Infection from blood products and unsterilized needles is a possible cause, but probably accounts for a very small proportion of cases. Transmission by flies, mosquitoes, or other insects does not appear important. Educational efforts have advocated the following measures: limiting the number of sexual partners, use of condoms, changing methods of intercourse, screening transfused blood to prevent the use of infected products, sterilization of needles, promotion of the use of disposable needles, among others. Educational efforts have resulted in a marked change in sexual habits at least among the homosexual population of San Francisco (Anonymous, 1987).

*   *   *

The 20 categories of disease listed above appear to be the leading causes of ill health and death globally. The relative importance within an individual country, region, district, or neighborhood can also vary, as discussed in the next section. As is evident from these descriptions, the available knowledge does indicate some directions and interventions that can allay disease and disability. Further study and innovation are still needed to identify the best methods for application and utilization of this knowledge in the field to ensure that a reasonable impact ensues from the health promotion efforts. Several conditions, namely respiratory infections, low birth weight, and injuries, require greater basic and epidemiologic research to develop and evaluate better control measures.

Analysis of Burden at the Local Level

Tables 1 and 2 (pp. 4 and 15) present the global estimates of burden of illness. Planners may find, however, that they need to develop comparable lists for an entire nation, region, district, community, or even a neighborhood. Before data collection, planners should consider their needs and the potential uses for the data. Ideally, one should concentrate on collecting and verifying the data on the burden of illness for those diseases that can be efficaciously, easily, and, cheaply treated or prevented. As a group, these usually include the infectious diseases that are controllable through application of an array of immunologic and therapeutic techniques. For example, information on cancer or diabetes may be interesting but less valuable, as little action can be taken to control these conditions if the enviroment remains desperately poor.

If not already compiled within the local health division, the data required for health system planning may be sought through a variety of governmental or private organizations and institutions. Several sources include: (1) present reporting system, (2) population surveys, (3) hospital and clinic records, (4) vertical programs, (5) sources outside the governmental health services, and (6) surveillance systems.

• *Present Reporting System.* In essentially all countries, some data have already been collected by health workers from the self-selected population that utilizes the health centers or subcenter facilities. Some of this information may also be transmitted to the district, regional, provincial, and or national level. However, numbers of cases reported through these methods should be viewed with skepticism, unless one can assure the accuracy of the diagnosis and completeness of the data. Factors limiting the reliability of this information include: lack of uniform case definition, limited reporting of cases (*i.e.,* only those cases that lie within the purview of the governmental health centers and hospitals), possible exclusion of cases handled or treated by other practitioners, failures or delays in transmission of data to central authorities, and varying enthusiasm to report a disease. As a result, the reported cases may represent underreporting or overreporting, and may minimize or aggrandize the numbers of cases actually occurring.

For example, serologic surveys indicate that, in areas without measles vaccine, practically all individuals have had the disease by adolescence. In contrast, only a small number of these large number of cases are reported annually. WHO reported that 13 neonatal tetanus surveys and 13 poliomyelitis surveys in various countries revealed that routine surveillance systems generally have marked deficiencies enumerating only between 1% and 26% of the cases actually occurring (Weekly Epidemiological Record, 1982). To obtain accurate information on disease occurrence, these data should be supplemented from other sources mentioned below.

- *Surveys of the Population.*   More accurate determinations of disease incidence and prevalence can be obtained, but at a greater cost in terms of manpower and other resources. Before embarking on a survey, a planner should consider several questions: Will better estimates change program or policy? Is there a good survey tool? Can the system cope with the extra effort of the survey and subsequent programmatic changes that may occur as a consequence of the survey findings? The type of survey performed can influence the completeness of the assessment of incidence and prevalence. For example, in a comparison of the estimated incidence of poliomyelitis by three survey methods in different regions of the Cameroon, house-to-house survey in a rural area demonstrated a higher incidence than did a survey of school children (Heyman, *et al.*, 1983; LaForce, *et al.*, 1980). The WHO/EPI developed a standardized cluster sampling method for evaluating immunization uptake, but increasingly, this format has been applied in surveys of other diseases (Henderson and Sundarsen, 1982; Malison, *et al.*, 1987; Rothenberg, *et al.*, 1985). A cheaper, faster method called Lot Quality Assessment Sampling (LQAS), which is based upon quality control techniques developed in light bulb manufacturing, is under field testing in several areas of the world. The Pan American Health Organization (PAHO) and the United States National Academy of Sciences through the Bureau of Science and Technology in Development (NAS/BOSTID) together fund the investigations of the Centers for Disease Control, the Costa Rican government, the Harvard School of Public Health, and the Peruvian government.

Carefully conducted surveys are a powerful tool for determining the incidence and prevalence of various diseases, risk factors, and other parameters, but require careful planning and may require substantial manpower to ensure accurate and usable collection of information.

• *Hospital and Clinic Records.* Hospital and clinic visitors represent a biased population (*i.e.,* those who can afford the time and money to travel to and pay for care). Usually, only those who live within a short distance (two to five kilometers) of these facilities actually utilize their services. Other factors affecting utilization and consequently completeness of the records as measures of disease occurrence include: population density; proximity of other hospitals, clinics and other practitioners; and cost of care. Hospital and outpatient records and clinic visits may also be used for evaluating the effectiveness of interventions targeted for particular population groups. For example, if pregnant women were identified for a specific health program, a review of the age, sex, and other characteristics of the patients seen in the hospital or clinic may reveal whether this high-risk group is receiving care. The occurrence of measles, pertussis, or poliomyelitis cases would denote the failure of an immunization program.

• *Vertical Programs.* Prior or current vertical or categorical programs aimed at control of particular diseases, such as mobile programs, should provide information on the incidence or prevalence of the particular disease in various regions and on seasonality.

• *Sources Outside the Governmental Health System.* These include donor agencies which have studied or instituted programs in particular regions or localities, investigators at medical schools, and veterinary institutions (especially for zoonoses such as leishmaniasis, trypanosomiasis, rabies, and plague). Although these programs work with the approval and consent of the government, they work in parallel and may not efficiently share data.

• *Surveillance Systems.* An effective surveillance system for ongoing reporting and collecting of information requires some definition of priorities. The reporting and recording system must be as short and as simple as possible to encourage participation by busy health workers. Only essential decision-making data should be collected and, in recording the information, should follow standardized case definitions. Regular reporting and feedback, that is, distribution and publication of the data collected and response, will encourage careful habits.

In addition to routine reporting systems, sentinel site surveillance and community diagnosis systems have been used for monitoring, particularly in the efforts to expand immunization coverage. Sentinel posts are chosen to represent health facilities of the geographic area under surveillance and should include both urban and rural localities. The posts should include areas suspected to have problems with program implementation in order to monitor the worst situation. The most important consideration is willingness of the facility authorities and personnel to participate, existence of reasonable record keeping, and an adequate volume of patients (Dondero, 1983).

Community diagnosis involves the population-based monitoring of health events rather than selection of those events occurring at the specific sentinel health facilities. Its foundation consists of an annual census plus regular reporting of health events by the community health or other workers during their routine visits to all homes in a carefully defined neighborhood. Save the Children Foundation and the Jamkhed Comprehensive Rural Health Project, among others, have successfully used illiterate community members for this task and for encouraging participation in immunization and health education programs, since these individuals know everyone in the appropriate target group. This system helps alert village inhabitants to the most important health problems and sensitizes them to the control efforts.

The data on births, deaths, diseases, and other health events under surveillance are aggregated centrally. One drawback is the dependence of disease diagnosis and attribution of cause of death to these community health workers unless the system makes special arrangements to follow-up and more accurately determine the causes of morbidity and mortality. This system has been used successfully in programs in Haiti; Narangwal, Jamkhed, and Ludhiana, India; Matlab, Bangladesh; Kasongo, Zaire; and several other countries (Berggren, *et al.*, 1981; Parker, *et al.*, 1978; The Kasongo Project Team, 1981). Several methods exist for collecting accurate data and estimating disease incidence and prevalence. Special attention should be given to identifying high-risk population groups. Reliable information systems, which include ongoing monitoring and surveillance, are key elements for health service planning, management, and evaluation. In many existing health systems, inadequate attention has been accorded to the establishment of reliable, timely evaluation and surveillance, which has resulted in lack of documentation of the impact of health services and lack of the information needed to assure good management, administration, and quality control.

Available Interventions

For each of the diseases and conditions listed in Table 2 (p. 15), a variety of preventive and therapeutic measures has been tried, yielding a range of results. Some control methods have been more successful than others in preventing illness and curing disease. Few possess highly efficacious, long-lasting, inexpensive, technically feasible control methods that can be easily employed in all parts of the world. Immunizations are among the best available, and even these require a more extensive, well-organized management and distribution system than initially imagined to assure sustained provision to the high-risk groups.

Table 7 provides the efficacy of available preventive interventions and Table 8, the therapeutic interventions for the conditions presented in Table 2, along with some estimates of costs. *Efficacy* measures the proportional decline in death and disease incidence or prevalence in a clinical trial of the given method. For example, there is a 90% decline in measles incidence among those vaccinated compared to those unvaccinated when all are exposed in an outbreak. Efficacy is measured in an experimental situation in which special efforts are made to assure proper administration, provision, and patient or client compliance. This distinguishes the results of an efficacy study from those found in the usual conditions of health systems, in which less care and concentration can be spent on coverage, technique, and compliance. The health *impact* of a given intervention in the field is determined by: (1) efficacy of the intervention, (2) ability to identify the appropriate risk group, (3) coverage, (4) provider compliance, and (5) patient or client compliance (Tugwell, *et al.*, 1986). These are defined as follows:

1.   *Efficacy.* The evaluation of the efficacy of an intervention assumes ideal conditions. If the intervention will avert only a small number of deaths or cases of disease under optimal conditions, it will avert even fewer when applied to an open population.

2.   *Screening and diagnostic accuracy.*   In statistical terms, diagnostic accuracy is the sensitivity (ability) of the patient or provider to diagnose a particular disease, condition, or target group. If the method or criteria used for diagnosis has a low sensitivity or poor accuracy, then many target individuals who might benefit from the preventive or curative interventions would be missed. Specificity is the ability to recognize that other conditions are not, in fact, the particular disease under attention. A low specificity would cause control measures to be initiated inappropriately, adding unnecessary cost, and possibly incurring an adverse impact on health if the treatment has side effects.

3.   *Health provider compliance.*   The health provider must have adequate training and provide the health practice correctly. For example, the instructor must correctly teach the mother how to prepare and administer a home-based oral rehydration solution before she can appropriately use it. The health worker must correctly instruct clients in the use of condoms or birth control pills or screens and netting (for repelling insects) before these can have any effect.

4.   *Patient compliance.*   In the case of oral rehydration therapy (ORT), adequate provision of the therapy would involve appropriate mixing to attain the right dilution of salt, sugar, and water or a properly mixed ORT packet. It would also involve the correct administration of the solution to a child with diarrhea. In the case of family planning practices, the birth control pills must be ingested daily or condoms worn in the correct manner and at the appropriate time.

5.   *Coverage.*   Coverage refers to the extent to which the efficacious maneuver, procedure, or services are appropriately utilized by all those who would benefit from them. Coverage differs from patient compliance; coverage describes whether the individual makes contact with the health professional, and patient compliance refers to the adherence of the patient to the subsequent advice received. Each of these factors will influence the community effectiveness or health impact of a particular program (Tugwell *et al.*, 1986).

If the health impact is less than expected, each of these factors should be evaluated. For example, if your surveillance system reports that diarrheal deaths continue to occur frequently in spite of an ORT program, one might investigate and evaluate how the health workers define diarrhea. (This will affect when they begin

Table 7.   Efficacy of Preventive Measures

DISEASE	PREVENTIVE MEASURE	EFFICACY[1] (%)	COST[2] ($)
Respiratory Infections			
Pneumococcus	vaccine (23 valent)	25-60	5+/dose
H. influenza B[3]	vaccine	*	10+/dose
Influenza virus A&B	vaccine	80	10+/dose
	chemoprophylaxis (amantadine)	50-80	10/dose
Measles	vaccine (EPI)	90	0.06/dose
Pertussis	vaccine (EPI)	63-95	0.02/dose
Diptheria	vaccine (EPI)	90	0.02/dose
Unspecified pathogen	change cooking stoves[4]	*	2
	decrease smoking[4]	*	*
	decrease low birth weight[4]	*	*
	improve housing[4]	*	*
	vitamin A[4]	*	<0.05/dose
Low Birth Weight	malaria prophylaxis	0-70	<1
	antenatal care	50	10+
	nutritional supplements	-20 to 50	10+
	education	*	*
Circulatory System	Aspirin	0-20	1-2
	Control hypertension	20	30+
	Reduce fat intake	0-25	30+
Diarrheal Diseases			
Cholera	vaccine	30-60	1
Toxigenic *E. coli*	vaccine	under trial	*
Rotavirus	vaccine	under trial	*
Salmonella	water & sanitation[11]	0-60	2-46[5]
Shigella	water & sanitation	50	2-46[5]
Unspecified cause	water & sanitation	20-50	2-46[5]
	measles vaccine	10	0.06/dose
	prevention of low birth weight	*	*
	nutritional supplements	0-25	10+
	hygiene	20-50	*
	vitamin A	*	<0.05/dose
Measles	vaccine (EPI)	90	0.06
Injuries	modified cooking fires	*	*
Malnutrition	nutrition education	0-50	2+
	nutritional supplements	0-50	10+
Neoplasms[6]	vaccine (HBsAg)	under trial	1/dose
	periodic examinations	10-50	1+
Malaria	mosquito control (insecticides, larvicides, environmental management, netting)	30-90	2+
	chemoprophylaxis	0-80	<0.02/dose
	vaccine	under trial	*

Table 7.   (cont.)

DISEASE	PREVENTIVE MEASURE	EFFICACY (%)	COST ($)
Tetanus	vaccine	90	0.02/dose
	TBA training	40-60	*
Tuberculosis	vaccine (EPI)	0-80	0.10/dose
	active case identification	30-50	*
	chemoprophylaxis	70-80	1-2
Hepatitis B	vaccine	80	1/dose
Whooping cough	vaccine	80	0.02/dose
Typhoid	vaccine	50-60	2-5
Maternal Mortality	family planning	*	*
	TBA training	*	*
	rapid referral	*	*
	local delivery facilities	*	*
Meningitis			
Neisseria	vaccine (A,C,Y,W135)	60-90	10 + /dose
	chemoprophylaxis	70	1
Pneumococcal	vaccine	*	5 + /dose
H. influenza B	vaccine	0-80[7]	10 + /dose
	chemoprophylaxis	0-80	1
Schistosomiasis	chemotherapy[8]	70-90	1 +
	mollusk control	30	1-3
	water & sanitation	0-25	2-46
Syphilis	condoms	*	*
	education	*	*
Amebiasis	water & sanitation	25	2-46
	hygiene	*	*
Chagas Disease	housing[9]	*	100 +
	insecticide[9]	*	5 +
	nets[9]	*	2
Rheumatic Fever & Heart Disease	chemotherapy	50 +	1 +
Hookworm	water & sanitation	50	2-46
	footwear	low	*
Rabies	vaccine	60 +	*
Diphtheria	vaccine	90 +	0.02/dose
HIV (AIDS)	education	*	*
Dengue	mosquito control	0-90	*
Hepatitis A	water & sanitation	*	2-46
	hygiene	*	*
	immune globulin	60-80	1 +
Yellow fever	vaccine	90	<1
Japanese B encephalitis	vaccine	60-80	*
Ascariasis	water & sanitation	*	2-46
	chemotherapy-mass	60-75	1
Giardiasis	water & sanitation	0-50	2-46

Table 7. Efficacy of Preventive Measures (cont.)

DISEASE	PREVENTIVE MEASURE	EFFICACY (%)	COST ($)
Poliomyelitis	vaccine	80-90	0.03/dose[10]
Leprosy	vaccine (BCG)	20-60	0.10/dose
	active case identification	50	1-2
	chemoprophylaxis	0-80	0.50
Leishmaniasis	animal and sand fly control	30-90	1-2
Trichuriasis	water & sanitation	50	2-46
	chemotherapy	60+	1
Filariasis	mosquito control	60-95	.50-3
	chemotherapy	50-90	5
	screens & nets	*	*
Dracunculiasis	protected water	90+	2
Onchocerciasis	simulium control	90	20+
	chemotherapy	under trial	0
	nodulectomy	poor	*
African trypanosomiasis	fly control	80	*
	chemoprophylaxis	80	*
	surveillance and treatment	*	2-4
Unspecified Infant & Child Mortality	vitamin A	20-30	<0.05/dose
	child spacing	0-50	*

1. Efficacy measures the proportional decline in incidence or prevalence of the disease in carefully performed trials of the interventions. When any intervention is utilized in an open population, its actual effectiveness in preventing disease will be less because compliance is not good. Some of the interventions are single-dose vaccines (measles) while others require multiple dose (DTP) or continual administration (*e.g.*, aspirin to prevent heart attacks, a form of circulatory disease). Still others require initial investment in an environmental change and then continued maintenance (*e.g.*, water and sanitation).

2. Cost estimates are for single doses of vaccines or short courses of drugs. Annualized costs are estimated for items requiring long-term maintenance, such as water and sanitation or long-term drugs. Cost of delivery system is not included in these estimates.

3. *Hemophilus influenza B* does prevent meningitis in infants more than 18 months of age, but these studies have not examined the incidence of respiratory disease. The studies were performed in the North, where Hemophilus respiratory disease is relatively rare.

4. These measures have not yet been tested in field trials to measure efficacy.

5. Annualized cost of water ranges from $2/capita for drilling wells with handpumps in rural areas to more than $20/capita in some densely populated urban areas. Annualized cost of sanitation ranges from $4 for rural latrines to $26 for urban sewerage.

6. Hepatitis B hepatocellular carcinoma probably can be prevented by vaccine; however, this agent is under trial. Periodic Pap smears for cervical cancer, breast exams, mammography, stool blood, etc., can identify precancerous or cancerous cells at an early stage if performed regularly.

7. Vaccine induces immunity only in children older than 18 months.

8. Chemotherapy probably must be repeated every few months to prevent disease.

9. Long-term efficacy of these interventions is unknown, as disease takes many years to develop.

10. Triple valent oral polio vaccine costs 2 cents/dose; inactivated polio vaccine costs 50 cents/dose.

11. The range of efficacy represents the results of several different studies.

*   is no data.   TBA is traditional birth attendant.

Table 8.   Efficacy of Therapeutic Measures

DISEASE	TREATMENT	EFFICACY[a] (%)	COST[b] ($)
Acute Lower Respiratory Infections			
Pneumococcus & *H. influenza B*	antibiotics	90	0.08-20[1]
Influenza	amantadine	60	1-5
Respiratory syncytial virus	ribavarine	60	100 +
Whooping cough	antibiotics	50-75	1
Diphtheria	antibiotics plus antitoxin	90	1-5
Unspecified pathogen	antibiotics	35-82	.08-.20[1]
Circulatory System	chemotherapy	—[2]	10 +
Low Birth Weight	nutrition & support	—[3]	*
Diarrheal Diseases	ORT[4]	50-90	0.01-1.0
Measles	—[9]	—	—
Injuries	first aid	—[3]	*
Malnutrition	nutrition and education	0-50	2 +
Neoplasms	chemotherapy	low[5]	100 +
	surgery	low[5]	100 +
	radiation	low[5]	100 +
Malaria	chemotherapy	90	0.10-5
Tetanus	hospital care	65	100 +
Tuberculosis	chemotherapy[6]	80	10-100
Hepatitis B	—	—	—
Whooping cough	antibiotics	50-75	1
Typhoid	chemotherapy	90	1
Maternal Mortality[7]			
Sepsis	chemotherapy	60-90	10 +
Hemorrhage	transfusion & surgery	90	100 +
Obstructed labor	surgery	60 +	100 +
Eclampsia	chemotherapy	90[3]	10 +
Meningitis	chemotherapy	80 +	1
Schistosomiasis	chemotherapy	90	1-5
Syphilis	chemotherapy	90	0.20 +
Amebiasis	chemotherapy	60 +	2
Chagas Disease	chemotherapy	poor	—
Rheumatic Fever	chemotherapy	50	1
Hookworm	chemotherapy	90	1
Rabies	—[10]	—	—
Diphtheria	antibiotics plus antitoxin	90	1-5
HIV (AIDS)	chemotherapy	under trial	100 +

Table 8. Efficacy of Therapeutic Measures (cont.)

DISEASE	TREATMENT	EFFICACY[a] (%)	COST[b] ($)
Dengue	—[9]	—	—
Hepatitis A	—[9]	—	—
Yellow fever	—[9]	—	—
Japanese B encephalitis	—[9]	—	—
Ascariasis	chemotherapy	90 +	1
Giardiasis	chemotherapy	90	1
Poliomyelitis	—[9]	—	—
Leprosy	chemotherapy[11]	90	5-25
Leishmaniasis	chemotherapy	poor	—
Trichuriasis	chemotherapy	90	1
Filariasis	chemotherapy	under trial	—
Dracunculiasis	chemotherapy	poor	—
Onchocerciasis	chemotherapy	under trial	0[12]
African trypanosomiasis	chemotherapy	poor	—

[a]*Efficacy* —measures the likelihood of cure of disease in carefully performed trials. When any intervention is applied to an open population, its actual effectiveness in preventing disease will be less because compliance may not be as good. Some of the interventions can cure (*e.g.*, antibiotics) but other interventions can only decrease the rate of disease progression (drugs for circulatory system diseases).

[b]*Cost* —estimates a short course of drugs. For those that must be maintained over many years, an annualized cost is estimated. For drugs, cost of delivery system is not included.

1. Outpatient antibiotics cost $0.08 to $0.40 per course. Inpatient antibiotics cost $0.50 to $20.00 per course.
2. Chemotherapy improves, but does not cure the disease. The individual must continue to take medication for many years. Annual cost of drugs is high.
3. Cost and efficacy depend on severity of illness.
4. Oral rehydration therapy.
5. Anticancer drugs, surgery, and/or radiation can cure only a small number of cancers. More frequently, they temporarily palliate the symptoms. All are expensive.
6. Tuberculosis chemotherapy must continue for at least 6 months.
7. The major causes of maternal mortality are post-partum hemorrhage and sepsis. Treatment requires hospitalization and is quite successful if treatment begins early. Cost of hospital care depends on severity of illness and location.
8. Chemotherapy prolongs the life of patients with AIDS but does not cure.
9. No specific treatment is available for this disease, only supportive care and treatment of complications as needed.
10. No treatment; mortality is essentially 100%.
11. Leprosy chemotherapy must continue for at least 1 year, and frequently many years.
12. Merck, Sharpe, and Dohme provides ivermectin free through the WHO.

ORT and when they instruct mothers to begin ORT); how the health workers use ORT themselves and teach mothers to mix and use it; how well the mothers mix and administer ORT to children; what proportion of the population is covered by the ORT program. The efficacy in averting dehydration and death has been fairly well established in community settings (Egemen and Bertan, 1980; Rowland and Coles, 1980; Watkinson and Watkinson, 1982). In another example, if vaccine preventable diseases continue to occur despite supposedly high acceptance of immunization, one might evaluate the potency of the vaccine, the ability of the health workers to identify the children who would benefit from immunization, the method health workers follow to store, carry, dilute, and administer the material, and the comprehension of mothers and families regarding the importance of vaccines and compliance when requests are made to bring their children in to receive treatment.

When planning health services, the priority interventions should be efficacious, inexpensive, feasible, and targeted at controlling those diseases that cause the greatest morbidity and mortality. Priority does not imply exclusivity, as other interventions may be accorded importance for other reasons by administrators or by the community. For example, all individuals want ready access to first aid and curative care. Nevertheless, a health system with the goal of trying to reduce illness and death as rapidly and efficiently as possible should, at least, provide those interventions capable of efficiently averting the most disease, to the group most in need and most likely to benefit.

Table 9 presents the efficacious short-term control measures that can be provided through health systems. The choice among these measures is often limited by local disease and health resources, since some of the interventions are fairly expensive. Other possible interventions and determinants of health status are discussed in the section *Determinants of Health* (p. 50). The global priorities for implementation in health-promoting programs is addressed in Chapter 4.

The identification of global health research priorities also begins by examining and comparing Table 2 (Causes of Death, p. 15) with Table 7 (Efficacy of Preventive Measures p. 43) and Table 8 (Efficacy of Therapeutic Measures, p. 46). Biomedical and basic research appears key for those conditions causing substantial disease and death for which no or only expensive interventions are available.

Table 9. Efficacious Short-Term Control Measures*

DISEASE	PREVENTION	CURE
Respiratory Disease		
Pneumococcus	—	chemotherapy
H. influenza	—	chemotherapy
Measles	vaccine	—
Whooping cough	vaccine	—
Diphtheria	vaccine	—
Diarrheal Disease		
Rotavirus	—	oral rehydration
Toxigenic *E. Coli*	—	oral rehydration
Cholera	—	oral rehydration
Measles	vaccine	—
Malaria	—	chemotherapy
Tetanus	vaccine	—
Hepatitis B	vaccine	—
Whooping Cough	vaccine	—
Meningitis		
Pneumococcus	—	chemotherapy
H. influenza	chemoprophylaxis	chemotherapy
N. meningitidis		
(A,C,Y,W135)	vaccine	chemotherapy
	chemoprophylaxis	—
Schistosomiasis	chemotherapy	chemotherapy
Syphilis	—	chemotherapy
Amebiasis	—	chemotherapy
Hookworm disease	chemotherapy	chemotherapy
Diphtheria	vaccine	—
Yellow Fever	vaccine	—
Ascariasis	chemotherapy	chemotherapy
Trichuriasis	chemotherapy	chemotherapy
Filariasis	chemotherapy	chemotherapy
Dracunculiasis	protected water	—

*Preventive or curative measures that are at least 60% efficacious in field trials, require 7 days or less of compliance, and can be provided through established health services. If field trails have resulted in a wide range of efficacy, as in the case of BCG vaccine for the prevention of tuberculosis, then it is not listed. For water supplies, the new hand pump developed by the UNDP/World Bank program requires minimal maintenance.

For those common diseases for which interventions are available but result in limited health impact, research may be needed at various levels: (1) at the engineering or development stage to improve delivery systems or to identify a cheaper maneuver; or to discover a less expensive, more sensitive and specific diagnostic tool; (2) at the operations or health services research level to improve the training of health workers and their compliance, to improve patient knowledge and compliance, or to improve management systems.

Oral polio vaccine presents an example of this phenomenon. In the North, polio incidence essentially disappeared as a result of widespread use of polio vaccine. In some populations in developing countries, however, use of the vaccine induces a lower concentration of serum antibodies than usually is found among vaccinees in the North. Efforts are under way to try to improve the immunogenicity of the vaccines. Malaria control presents another example in which efficacious measures have had less impact on disease prevalence than expected.

Social Benefits of Control Measures

Many of the control measures listed in Tables 7 and 8 reduce disease and disability, in addition to delivering substantial benefits to other sectors of society. Water and sanitation are outstanding examples, as these conveniences not only decrease diarrheal disease, typhoid illness and death, but also, and possibly more importantly, decrease the time spent (primarily by women) in drawing water, and provide water for irrigation, agriculture, and animal husbandry. Education of women, and to a lesser extent of men, affects health, fertility, and agricultural productivity (Caldwell, 1979; Cochran, 1980 and 1986; United Nations, 1985). Family planning reduces maternal morbidity and mortality, improves child survival through longer birth intervals, yields greater infant birth weights and older onset of childbearing, and decreases population growth. Benefit-cost analysis is one method for weighing the costs and benefits accrued in other sectors of society from a given program or project, but without comparing specific models, one cannot weigh the relative benefits of different interventions.

Determinants of Health

Health, as broadly defined in the Alma Ata Declaration, is a state of well-being which permits an individual to lead a socially and economically productive life. Health results from the intermingling of a number of factors. The schema in Figure 3 presents these various factors and provides a framework for considering alternative strategies for health improvement (Barnum and Barlow, 1984; Mosley and Chen, 1984; PAHO, 1986). The figure attempts to over-

Figure 3.   Determinants of Health

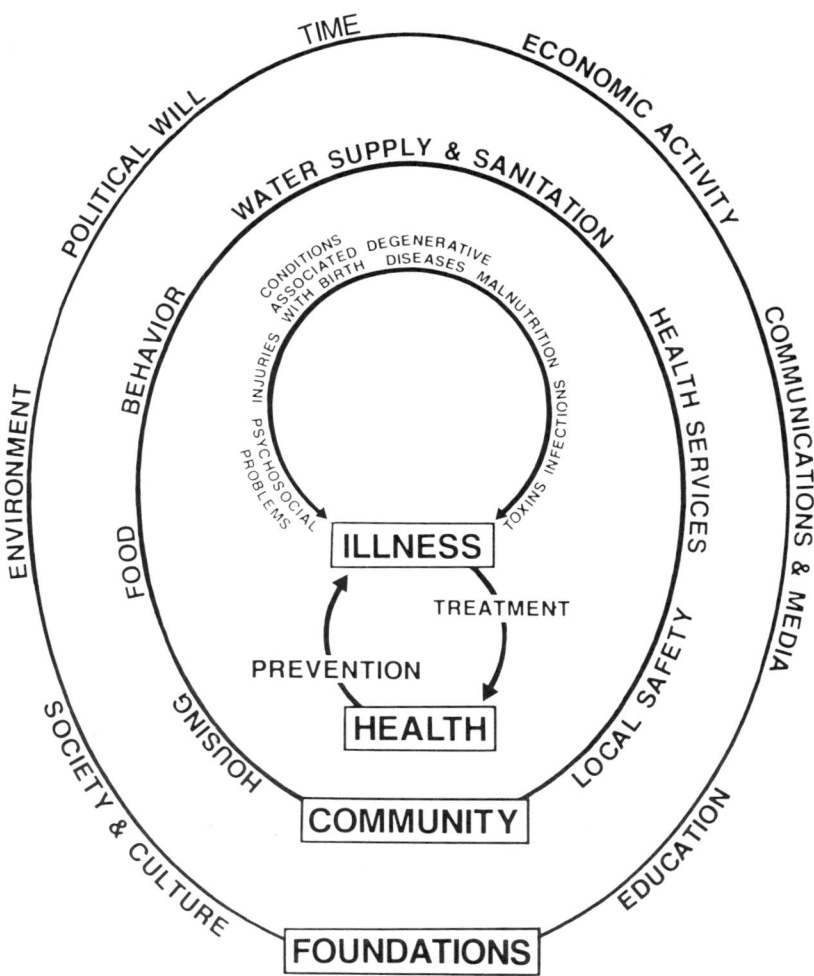

come the narrow view of many health professionals who feel that provision of specific health interventions comprises the only (or necessarily the best) way to improve well-being. It also attempts to balance the view that health improvement results primarily from social and economic improvement (McKeown, 1976). All these salient features affect health and eventually operate through the immediate ailments identified in the inner ring. In formulating strategies to improve health, careful analysis of specific situations and weighing of possible alternatives (behavior change, infectious disease control, curative care, increasing food supply, education) may lead to the conclusion that a combined approach involving a number of activities from a spectrum of sectors may provide the most effective means to good health.

All of the determinants listed in Figure 2 operate by either preventing illness and maintaining health, or by treating illness and restoring health. Certainly, prevention is preferable. They are divided into three levels:

1.   The first level (inner ring) pertains to the *Illnesses* that represent the direct causes of sickness and loss of health: malnutrition, infectious diseases, degenerative diseases, and so forth.

2.   The second level (middle ring) details the factors operating within the *Community* which modify, through prevention or alleviation, the diseases and conditions of the first level: status of health services, access to water and sanitation, and so on.

3.   The third level (outer ring) represents the societal or cultural determinants of health which form the basis or *Foundation* for the other two levels. Changes in societal factors modify factors at the community level, which, in turn, affect the prevention or treatment of first level ailments. For example, increasing the political will to improve health leads to the appropriation of more resources for building health centers, hiring and training health workers, stocking drugs, and vector control.

Since there is abundant interaction amongst the components of all three levels, no attempt is made to separate the components at each level. The figure highlights the intersectoral origins of health, underscoring the concept that improvements in health may most efficiently or sustainably occur by adjustments in elements at either the Community or Foundation levels rather than just improvements in health systems or development of new technologies for prevention and cure of individual illnesses.

Description of the Components (Figure 2)

- *Diseases and Conditions (Illnesses).* These are presented in the innermost circle and are modified, treated, or prevented by factors in the outer two rings representing the Community and Foundation levels. Examples of specific conditions in each category are given below:

Malnutrition—includes deficiencies in required nutrients such as vitamin A and D, iodine, and protein energy, as well as excesses, such as overconsumption of fats and calories.

Degenerative diseases—include atherosclerotic cardiovascular diseases (heart attacks) and neoplasms or cancers. An increasing number of cancers seem to have multiple causation. For example, the toxins in tobacco induce lung cancers in individuals with genetic predisposition, and hepatitis B virus can induce hepatic cancers in a small percentage of those who are long-term virus carriers. Most of these degenerative diseases have no specific prevention or cure but treatment can slow the progression of disease.

Toxins—include occupational exposures such as to asbestos, and environmental exposures such as to aflatoxin and ciguaratoxin in fish, pesticides, or tobacco smoke.

Infections—in most instances are the most common, easily prevented and treated cause of disability and death in the developing countries. In addition to the infectious diseases found in industrialized countries (*e.g.,* respiratory tract infections, diarrheas, and immunization-preventable infections) this category includes diseases unique to warm climates (malaria, filariasis. etc.) and a great variety of microorganisms, most of which require specific methods for prevention and cure: viruses, bacteria, protozoa, helminths, among others.

Injuries—are rapidly becoming one of the most important causes of illness throughout the world, particularly as they affect young adults. Injuries include occupational injuries, motor vehicle and household accidents, among others.

Conditions associated with birth—comprise the genetically related conditions, congenital defects, and illnesses associated with pregnancy that involve both the mother and the infant: for example, low birth weight, preterm delivery, maternal morbidity, and mortality.

53

Psychosocial and mental illness—can affect many other diseases and independently result in substantial economic and social losses in terms of productive years of life. The advancements in drug treatment and psychological therapy allay only a part of the disability from these illnesses.

- *Community Determinants.*   These promote health and well-being by averting or alleviating the immediate problems of ill health listed in level one. In turn, these determinants are modified by the societal and foundational determinants of the outermost level.

Behavior—This feature includes smoking habits, diet, hygiene, compliance with health services, activities which influence contact with disease-transmitting vectors such as mosquitoes and flies, and an enormous number of other health-promoting or inhibiting activities. Communication and education can influence individual behavior, for example, by causing an individual to live in a more healthy manner by decreasing smoking or changing diet.

Two of the main constraints on healthful behavior are *time* and *knowledge.* If mothers have no time to care for and feed their families because of the necessity to spend many hours daily drawing water, grinding grain, and working in the fields, then the health of everyone in the household may suffer. Without knowledge of how to create health and without community, family, and societal reinforcement of these practices, healthy behaviors simply do not occur. Many of the other determinants presented at the community and foundation level influence the availability of time and knowledge.

Health Services—Numerous features affect the ability of primary health care services and referral hospitals to prevent or treat the illnesses mentioned above. These include accessibility; quality and quantity of health workers and facilities; financing patterns; technology available for diagnosis, treatment, and prevention; family planning services; and compliance, among others.

Water supply and sanitation—Some of the health mechanisms these facilities enhance include the following. Providing adequate quantities of water improves hygiene and increases crop yields and food supply and improves animal husbandry. Good quality water may decrease the spread of water-borne diseases. Appropriate use of sanitation facilities decreases fecally transmitted illnesses. Decreasing the time required to draw water will release mothers' time for childcare or household activities.

Housing—The rural or urban location of an individual's home, the type of construction, crowding, heat and energy sources, and ventilation all affect the diseases listed in the inner ring. Respiratory disease and Chagas disease present two clear examples. Pneumonias and bronchitis occur more commonly in crowded, poorly ventilated houses while transmission of Chagas disease requires the nesting of Reduviid bugs within the cracks and crannies frequently found in mud and thatch homes.

Environmental Safety—This component refers to the risk of injuries and toxic exposures in the environment, such as the type of cooking stove used in the home; the excreta disposal system in the home and its location; the safety of the area in which people work; the transport system used, which is particularly important as motor-vehicle accidents are a prime cause of injuries.

- *Determinants at the Foundation Level.*

Society and Culture—These have an enormous influence on individual health. Cultural tradition may encourage specific health-promoting and inhibiting behaviors, stimulate the use of health services and water and sanitation, determine the community response to mental illness, set societal structures for community leadership and role models, and regulate the role of women, to name only a few areas.

Economic Status—The economic status of the family and community affect all other determinants in the foundation, community, and disease condition levels. The desperately poor live without adequate food, housing, water and sanitation, hygiene, and access to health services.

Political Will—This component entails primarily the commitment or priority accorded to health at the family, community, regional, district, national, and international levels and the importance accorded to equity, that is, giving priority to services for the high-risk, most vulnerable and underserved groups which have the worst health status and greatest need. In several areas of the world, namely Sri Lanka, China, Costa Rica, and Kerala State, India, all of which have good health despite low average per capita income, the political will and desire for good health on the part of the people and government probably largely accounts for the surprisingly good health.

Ecology—The geographic location—desert, mountain, urban, rural (population density)—types of transport systems, need for irrigation, types of agriculture, and food availability all affect population health and well-being.

Education—Formal education has a substantial and lasting influence on health status. The level of literacy and educational attainment and equity of accessibility to education for men and women in all segments of society has substantial impact on health. Non-formal education is probably as important, but public health workers have only begun to recognize and exploit its potential. This area requires better delineation of appropriate methods.

Communication and Media—The types of media available (radio, TV, billboards, other marketing tools) influence how effectively the media can be used for health promotion. The communications revolution has already reached the villages of the world. Tiny villages in India have television and many households have radios. Stationary satellites allow simultaneous transmission of programs over an entire continent. TV and radio programs and commercials on breast-feeding, family planning, oral rehydration, and hypertension have educated people about healthy practices. Unfortunately, experience indicates that after a mass media campaign ends, people tend to go back to their old habits unless periodic short educational programs continue.

Time—In terms of both age and availability of leisure time, this determinant affects health in several different manners. The age at which an individual becomes ill influences long-term well-being and survival. The availability of time affects utilization of environmental safety measures, health services, and educational opportunities. Having enough spare time can affect a mother's ability to perform health-stimulating activities in the household.

Each of these determinants of health should be considered in developing and evaluating ways to improve well-being. Unfortunately, careful analysis of the effect of these determinants on health status is not available for most. One can only make reasonable estimates based on the circumstances in a given area. Despite the influence of so many factors on health status, for a number of conditions, specific health measures, such as vaccines and obstetric care to prevent maternal mortality, represent the most efficient means of control. For these, a disease-specific, health service delivery orientation may potentially have enormous impact.

3 *Research & Development*

Introduction

Achieving improved health involves the systematic application of existing knowledge and technologies to populations living in a variety of socio-economic and cultural settings. During the 20th century, a great transformation in health took place in the industrialized countries. The measures in large part responsible for this transformation included safe water supplies, sanitation, education (especially for women), personal hygiene, nutrition, immunizations, and specific therapies. The dramatic reduction in infant mortality in Costa Rica from 68/1000 in 1970 to 20/1000 in 1980 also seems secondary to these measures. However, the extension of primary health care would appear to be responsible for 40% of this reduction (Rosero-Bixby, 1986).

When all inhabitants of less developed countries have access to these facilities, health should improve. Yet, even these measures will not control all illness. Specific efforts are needed to find improved control measures for those diseases not yet curable or preventable and to assure their use by those at risk. The endeavor must involve the entire voyage, from discovery of an efficacious control measure, to development in the factory, and implementation at the village. The journey is often uncertain and prolonged. For new vaccines and drugs the time span from basic research and discovery, to development of the manufacturing process, through clinical trials and licensing, and finally, to availability for population-based utilization has taken up to 20 years. Fortunately, the new genetic and biomedical technologies afford a unique opportunity to shorten at least the time required to identify immunogens (vaccines) and synthesize them inexpensively (Martinez-Palomo, 1987).

With the twin goals of encouraging the effective utilization of available control measures and identifying new or improved preventive or treatment means, the priorities for research extend to many levels:

1.   Biomedical, laboratory-based efforts. These work toward the discovery of new interventions, such as vaccines or drugs, where none exist or the improvement of existing, relatively inefficacious, costly, or difficult-to-apply measures.

2.   Engineering and applied research. These try to facilitate distribution, such as improving the heat stabilization of products, simplifying administration procedures, modifying the manufacturing process, evaluating dosage schedules for drugs or vaccines, and studying innovative delivery schemes.

3.   Epidemiologic studies. These attempt to classify patterns of disease occurrence in human populations, test new diagnostic and preventive tools, and even more broadly, compare rates of occurrence of phenomena in various populations so as to increase understanding of the human situation.

4.   Operational and health systems research. This involves the methodical application of existing knowledge to varied socio-economic and cultural contexts. As described by Taylor (1984) (quoted below), health systems research emphasizes step-by-step improvement of services.

The innumerable obstacles and constraints that interfere with effective functioning need to be resolved in a progressive fashion through field studies. For every problem solved, others will emerge. This kind of continuing health system research can be an integral part of the health services.

---

5.   Social research. This covers economic, anthropologic, and intersectoral investigations including analysis of sources of be-

behavior, effects of education, agriculture, food supply, and nutrition; compliance, social mobilization; types of health-seeking behavior; costs of illness, and cost-effectiveness of intervention, water supplies, and sanitation.

Process for Analyzing Priorities

Priority topics for basic laboratory-based research include those causes of illness for which no adequate cure or prevention is presently recognized. An adequate intervention could be defined as one that is efficacious and easily provided within the present primary health care system with assurance of full compliance by those at risk. Vaccines and drugs requiring a minimal number of doses for long-term protection or cure are the prototype. However, vector control measures, micronutrient supplementation for nutritional deficiencies, and diagnostic and surveillance tools to identify those at risk and to insure compliance are also considered.

Table 9 presents the currently available interventions that have resulted in prevention or cure of 60% or more of the cases of disease with 7 doses (or visits) or less. Even compliance with short courses may be difficult. Delivering just 3 doses of DTP and polio vaccines to infants and children has frequently required nationwide and international mobilization. These interventions include: chemotherapy, vaccines, and oral rehydration.

Environmental changes, education, provision of new water supplies and sanitation do not appear on the list for several reasons. These control measures require persistent maintenance. Under study conditions, when well-functioning, carefully maintained water, sanitation, and environmental changes are present and usage is carefully reinforced and monitored, they can prevent 20% to 50% of a large variety of infectious diseases and conditions (Esrey, *et al.*, 1985; Esrey and Habicht, 1986). In contrast, under normal operating conditions, repair and usage usually decline along with health benefit. Education generally requires a prolonged effort and can affect many different conditions, but appears to have less than a 60% efficacy (Ashworth and Feachem, 1985; Clemens and Stanton, 1987; Feachem, 1984). Environmental change, education, water supplies, and sanitation all yield many benefits aside from health improvement. The list of short-term interventions in Table 9 (p. 49) is suprisingly short compared to Table 7 (p. 43) and Table

8 (p. 46) on the efficacy of therapeutic and preventive measures, which present a more complete and extensive list.

Those conditions without easily used, inexpensive, and efficacious interventions should be examined first in the evaluation of priorities for health research. If these diseases cause a substantial amount of disability, then application of successful control measures should improve health.

For evaluating priority areas for research at levels other than laboratory-based biomedical science, one can examine the present causes of death, identifying those that should be preventable with the known technology, and then analyze the constraints placed on their prevention. One can address the key questions:

1. Why are these deaths continuing to occur?
2. What are the limitations in the systems?
3. In what areas is further research necessary to overcome these constraints?

The answers may require local solutions or may uncover generic difficulties. Problem-solving requires detailed information about the system. An example might be diarrheal disease for which a combination of oral rehydration therapy, water supplies and sanitation, education, and some vaccines and drugs might be expected to essentially eliminate deaths from this disorder. As can be seen in Table 2 (p. 43), diarrhea is one of the most common causes of death and disease in the developing world. Yet, these interventions are not preventing deaths. The key areas for further study are:

1. determining the need (coverage and screening and diagnostic accuracy)
2. with operations research analyzing the constraints in local situations (health provider and patient compliance)
3. utilizing applied and engineering research to make the available interventions easier to use, and
4. identifying easier to use, more effective control measures.

Utilization and research needs must be clearly distinguished. When inexpensive, appropriate interventions are available, improving utilization is the priority. Nevertheless, ensuring health impact may require innovation, study, and problem-solving. Laboratory and engineering research becomes the priority when the control measures are inadequate. Priorities for implementation and utilization will be discussed later in Chapter 4.

Gaps in Interventions

Based on Table 2 (p. 43), which presents the major causes of death and Table 9 (p. 49), which presents the presently available efficacious interventions, Table 10 delineates the gaps; that is, those conditions for which no highly efficacious, inexpensive, simple, or technologically appropriate control strategies are available. For many of these conditions, control strategies exist but constraints to their application may include high cost, cultural incompatibility, complex technology, and marginal efficacy. These conditions include diarrheas, lower respiratory tract infections, malaria, injuries, maternal mortality, malnutrition, low birth weight, and tuberculosis among others. The status of the available control measures for diarrheal diseases has been carefully reviewed by the Control of Diarrheal Disease (CDD) program of the WHO and serves as an example of analysis for future research with other diseases.

Cases of diarrhea can be prevented through the use of soap and improved personal hygiene, provision of improved water supplies and sanitation, vaccines against specific organisms, breast-feeding, and prevention of low birth weight.

Deaths from diarrhea can be averted by using oral rehydration complemented by antibiotics in the relatively small proportion of cases caused by severe invasive organisms.

Behavior Change and Hygiene

The field studies of personal hygiene have measured reductions of between 14% and 48% in incidence rates when hands are washed regularly with soap (Feachem, 1984). Information is lacking on the optimal design of programs to improve personal hygiene. Certainly soap is inexpensive. In an area where community health workers already meet with family members, soap use could be encouraged. In an area with a successful social marketing system for family planning products and/or oral rehydration therapy, the system may easily be able to add soap to its product line. Costs and effectiveness of education programs to influence personal hygiene behavior are still unavailable (Stanton and Clemens, 1987). The long-term effectiveness of educational programs to change people's behavior has been disappointing. For example, in Bangladesh, a 1986 nation-wide evaluation of the diarrheal disease control status found that the massive efforts to educate people about oral rehydration have increased knowledge among more than

Table 10.   Conditions Lacking Simple, Short-Term, Efficacious Control Measures

Respiratory Diseases[1]

Diarrheal Disease[2]

Diseases of the Circulatory System

Low Birth Weight

Injuries

Malnutrition

Neoplasms

Tuberculosis

Typhoid

Maternal Mortality

Human Immunodeficiency Virus (HIV)(AIDS)

South American Trypanosomiasis

Rheumatic Fever and Heart Disease

Rabies

Dengue

Hepatis A

Japanese B Encephalitis

Giardiasis

Leprosy

Leishmaniasis

African Trypanosomiasis

1.   Acute respiratory infections from many of the bacteria can be cured with expeditious antibiotic treatment but the viral disease cannot.

2.   Although deaths from diarrheal disease appear preventable through liberal use of oral rehydration therapy, this does not allay the frequency and duration of disease. Invasive diarrheas, such as Shigella, usually require antibiotics for treatment.

90% of mothers and families, but a much smaller proportion used ORT at all, and an even smaller proportion used it appropriately. In another example, a Brazilian nation-wide campaign for promotion of breast-feeding resulted in a measurable increase that lasted only about a year. The evaluation concluded that educational efforts must be persistent to maintain an effect.

If people make behavioral changes without changing their internal values, beliefs, and attitudes, the new behaviors are less likely to continue when the external supports disappear. Most health promotion efforts have relied upon peer groups, social pressures, and even financial incentives to influence behavior. As soon as the peer group disappears or is no longer forced to behave in a certain way, the pressure is off the individual and he/she reverts back to his/her bad habits. To induce a persistent change in behavior requires an internal conversion to a belief that a given health behavior will affect him/herself, her/his own life. That is, there must be a belief in susceptibility. To induce this kind of change usually requires an individualized approach and is much harder, longer, and more difficult to accomplish than initially supposed.

Water and Sanitation

Water supplies and sanitation reduce diarrheal disease incidence by approximately 25% (Esrey and Habicht, 1986; Esrey, *et al.*, 1984). Low-cost, sturdy, low-maintenance water pumps are available, an outstanding achievement from years of careful field testing, research, and development on the part of the United Nations Development Programme/UNICEF/World Bank. These pumps, when correctly installed through accurately placed bore holes, provide substantial flows of water adequate for many families and can be centrally located for easy access. Depending on locations and depth of well, these can service 80 to 400 people per day with about 25 liters each of water. The initial costs are low because the pumps can be made locally and require minimal skilled maintenance. The same program has also tested and improved low cost sanitation technology (Cairncross, 1987). The amount of available water and the use of sanitation facilities seem to have a greater impact on diarrheal disease than the quality of available water (Feachem, *et al.*, 1978 and 1983). Improved water supplies directly benefit women by releasing time traditionally spent drawing water and also provide water for animal husbandry, irrigation for agriculture, and for cottage industries. Liberating women from the labor of seeking out water supplies means a greater amount of effort can be spent on more productive mother care or household activities.

Vaccines

The only presently available vaccine which prevents diarrheal disease is the measles vaccine. This prevents a small proportion of cases of diarrhea, but 10% or more of diarrhea deaths. These occur because severe diarrhea frequently follows measles (Feachem and Koblinsky, 1983). A child already weakened from the weight loss and complications of measles has an increased susceptibility for prolonged, complicated diarrhea. Rotavirus, cholera, and other vaccines are undergoing field testing at present. Cholera varies in incidence from country to country and even between locales within a country. Therefore, the vaccine may be of value only in high risk areas. In contrast, rotavirus diarrhea incidence among infants and toddlers, remains essentially the same throughout the world despite great variations in socio-economic and hygienic conditions. Therefore, a vaccine may be imperative to prevent transmission of the infection. At present, oral rehydration therapy can avert death from both diseases. Shigella and enterotoxigenic *E. coli* will likely have vaccines available within the next ten years.

Breast-feeding and Low Birth Weight

Promotion of breast-feeding of infants compared with bottle feeding reduces the incidence of diarrhea among babies younger than six months by at least 8% and deaths by about 25% (Feachem and Koblinsky, 1984). Prevention of low birth weight will avert a large proportion of infant deaths since it is such an overwhelmingly important determinant of infant and child health. For example, Ashworth and Feachem calculated that a 25% reduction in infant mortality would accrue from a fall in the prevalence of low birth weight from 30% to 15%. The diarrheal disease mortality could be expected to fall in parallel (Ashworth and Feachem, 1985).

Oral Rehydration

Oral rehydration has revolutionized the care of people with diarrhea by making treatment available in the home or outpatient clinic instead of only in hospitals. Many studies have demonstrated its effectiveness in the hospital, outpatient, community, and household setting. It is presently promoted through primary health care systems, family visits, media campaigns, social marketing, and other venues supported by nation-wide programs and international agencies. However, despite these massive, creative educational efforts, diarrheal disease mortality has not declined substantially. Increasing efforts to identify constraints in the programs and test solutions are needed. Much of these efforts require analysis of local situations and problem-solving operations research.

Antibiotics

Antibiotics are a mixed blessing for diarrhea. Their use shortens the course of illness for only a small proportion of cases, usually those caused by invasive organisms, such as Shigella and ameba. In general, antibiotics have been overused and prescribed as a panacea in place of the more time-consuming effort of instructing and overseeing the use of oral rehydration or because of a distrust in its efficacy. Changing the prescribing habits of physicians and other highly trained health workers may be one of the most difficult although cost-effective methods for reducing diarrheal deaths. The research needed for better diarrheal disease prevention spans several levels:

1.   Biomedical—vaccine and drug development particularly for organisms causing severe invasive disease;
2.   Applied and engineering—improving the content of ORT and its delivery, and continued refinement of excreta disposal facilities;
3.   Epidemiological—field trials of interventions, risk factors, and causes of low birth weight;
4.   Operations research—analysis and resolution of the constraints to effective use of ORT;
5.   Social research—culturally appropriate methods to promote personal hygiene, soap use, breast-feeding, and cost-effect analysis.

The other major conditions without excellent available interventions can be analyzed in a parallel fashion. However, before deducing priorities, the costs of research, likelihood of success, and funding levels must be considered and are addressed in the sections that follow.

Cost of Research

Research costs vary substantially depending on the topic involved and the type of research. Epidemiologic research requiring the continual monitoring of an extensive population tends to cost more than operations research limited to a more circumscribed area. Epidemiologic investigations can extend to multicenter studies in which centers in widely dispersed geographical locations use the same design, protocols, and measurement tools to evaluate the same problem simultaneously. Examples of such research endeavors include the World Fertility Survey; the multicenter study of infection during pregnancy and its affect on the outcome of pregnancy; the vitamin A, placebo-controlled field trials; and the typhoid, rotavirus, cholera, and leprosy vaccine field trials.

Examples of operations research to solve specific problems include: (a) developing within a primary health care system, a community financing scheme or revolving drug fund, (b) monitoring supervision methods and designing more effective formats, (c) identifying reasons for rapid turnover among community health workers and devising, applying, and evaluating possible solutions; (d) developing innovative training methods for faster learning and greater retention.

Applied research, such as (a) improving the manufacturing process for insecticides, drugs, and vaccines or (b) developing and testing a cold chain monitoring device, could be expected to be less expensive than extensive animal tests of prototype vaccines or drugs. The salient variables affecting cost are the number of individual investigators and other personnel, the proportion of their time spent on the project, location for the major research on the project (developing nation in Asia, Africa, Latin American, or Middle East, versus industrialized country), duration of the project, and capital expenditures for equipment and supplies.

The relative costs for some of these sample types of research are as follows. After identifying an efficacious immunogen in animal and preliminary human studies, vaccine development costs roughly $20 to $30 million and requires 7 to 10 years for testing and development (Institute of Medicine, 1984 and 1986). Operations research projects for primary health care administered by PRICOR, an organization funded through a contract from the USAID, cost an average of $54,000 in Africa, $74,000 in Asia, and $104,000 in Latin America. They lasted on average 20 months with a range of 4 to 36 months (Stinson, 1987; WHO, 1986). However, unlike biotechnical advances, operations research entails situation-specific problem-solving and testing of innovative solutions. The results tend to be applicable only locally; therefore, the studies must be repeated in many different sites.

An additional cost of the research not included in these estimates is the cost of administering the research funds, some of the technical assistance, and training for strengthening the capability of the local investigators and monitoring progress of the study.

The costs and length of time for vaccine development are so great because the process is complex. It involves large-scale human testing for side effects (reactogenicity), induction of measurable immunity (immunogenicity), and clinical trials followed by field trials for dose, efficacy, and streamlining of the manufacturing process (See Table 11).

The Ty21a typhoid vaccine trials present a good example of the obstacles that frequently occur in the process, providing the rationale for prolonged testing. The initial identification of the immunizing strain for typhoid occurred in 1975 (Germanier and Furer, 1975). Initial trials in Egypt induced a remarkably high protection. Subsequent trials in Chile using a modified dose and formulation (gelatin capsules and enteric-coated capsules instead of the initial liquid preparation used in Egypt) induced a much lower protection (22% to 59% in the first year compared with more than 80% in the original studies). In 1986, two more field trials began in Chile and Indonesia testing different formulations—a buffered liquid and enteric-coated capsules (WHO, 1986f).

Likelihood of Success

Not all research efforts automatically lead to an expected or clinically useful result. Even those investigations undertaken to streamline an engineering or manufacturing process, or to modify a product such as a handpump for a well, may not necessarily result in a better product within the budget and time-frame initially proposed. Basic or fundamental research projects may be undertaken with the goal of expanding knowledge in a particular sphere and building on the accumulating knowledge to eventually identify a clinically valuable tool or intervention. The years of fundamental work on genetics and immunology form the basis for the present biotechnological revolution, but these resulted in few applicable health products initially.

Table 11.   WHO Guidelines for Assessment of Malaria Vaccines.

Phase 0	Preclinical assessment of experimental vaccines to justify a first trial in man, and to support regulatory approval for such a trial.
Phase I	Trials in non-immune adult volunteers in non-endemic areas, to assess tolerability and immune responsiveness.
Phase II	Trials to demonstrate protective immunity against experimental challenge (IIA) and unquantified natural challenge (IIB).
Phase III	Assessment of vaccine efficiency against natural challenge in well-characterized trial areas, including populations with naturally acquired immunity.
Phase IV	Evaluation under field conditions of a licensed vaccine administered to a large population, to seek evidence of prevention of infection, and reduction in morbidity and mortality (sporozoite or merozoite vaccines) or reduction in transmission (gametocyte vaccines).

Note: Sporozoite and merozoite vaccines proceed through the four phases of testing. Gametocytes (or transmission blocking vaccines), which are not intended to induce protective immunity, proceed directly from Phase I to Phase IV.

Source: Perlman, 1986.

The factors involved in predicting probability of outcome include: present status of research and opportunities for advancement, expertise of the investigators, appropriateness of the budget (Does it include enough funds to pay for equipment and personnel?), "track-record" of the institution and scientists, facilities available at the institution and equipment needs included in the budget, logistics required for the research study, political climate, other commitments of the personnel involved, type of research, and the probability that a large population may benefit from the results.

Basic Research

Opportunities for rapid advancement exist in research at many levels. The biotechnological revolution provides an extraordinary opportunity to identify unique immunogens for vaccines, antigens for diagnosis and surveillance, and drugs (See p. 71 under Status of Research). Rapid methods exist for analyzing the metabolic pathways peculiar to invading organisms and synthesizing new drugs or vector control chemicals ("designer drugs") that will uniquely kill the pest but only minimally affect the metabolism of humans.

Among the infectious diseases of present paramount importance, research in acute respiratory diseases stands at a point similar to that of diarrheal diseases 10 or 15 years ago. Recent field trials demonstrating the success of short-term antibiotic treatment on morbidity and mortality can be compared to the discovery of oral rehydration for diarrheal disease. Vaccines against the major pathogens (pneumococcus, *Hemophilus influenzae*, influenza, respiratory syncytial virus, and others) are currently undergoing field trials. Research efforts should rapidly decrease the cost and increase the efficacy of these vaccines. Evaluation of innovative techniques for population-wide provision would appear to be next on the agenda.

Epidemiologic Research

Opportunities exist in analysis of risk factors and identification of future intervention strategies for diseases and conditions still not well-controlled in developing countries. Examples include sexually transmitted diseases, injuries, psychological and mental illness, field trials of the products of biotechnology research, and improved use of low-cost water pumps. Such studies will form the basis for future intervention strategies, but depend on local expertise for success.

Operations Research

Operations research may have a lower probability for success than other types of research. For several reasons, the findings may not immediately improve the efficiency or effectiveness of the primary health care system or of the provision of a given health intervention. For example, implementation of the findings may require a change in the bureaucracy and thus may be subject to political pressures. Or the research may address only one problem in the system, but other equally important problems may stand in the way. The Diarrheal Disease Control (CDD) Programme of WHO reviewed and evaluated 116 operational research projects which it had supported between 1978 and 1985. Only 22 projects yielded results that could be considered of high potential relevance for the operations of the Programme. Only 12 provided results that were actually used by the national CDD programme. As a consequence, the Programme is reorganizing and reconsidering its activities in this arena in order to make them more supportive or operational problem-solving (WHO, 1987).

The United States Agency for International Development (USAID) funded the Primary Health Care Operations Research Program (PRICOR). Upon termination of its operations research program for improving the functioning of Community Health Workers (CHW) the program concluded that it helped the investigators involved in the project to take into account the complex interactions and coequal importance of the three main ingredients: community health workers, community, and the health system in developing locally appropriate solutions. Input and involvement of these three ingredients were key for enhancing the feasibility and acceptability of solutions to complex problems. Nevertheless, the studies on CHW were often too long and involved too much data collection and analysis to rapidly yield results for management and decision-making. They found that although a study may identify and analyze a problem and suggest a solution, applying and evaluating that solution frequently were beyond the time-frame, budget, and scope of the project.

For example, a study in Nigeria addressed the problem of lack of supervision leading to low productivity of CHWs. As a result, strategies were recommended to the Federal and State Ministries of Health to improve training in supervisory methods and management techniques for current and future supervisory personnel. Also recommended were strategies to stress prevention and community outreach; to develop tools, guidelines, and protocols for use by the supervisors; and then to test these suggestions in the field. It took two years to reach this result, and it cost approximately $32,000, yet the ultimate relevance of the study based upon incorporation of the findings into the system and eventual improved CHW productivity is unclear.

In the PRICOR program, application of the solution was frequently beyond the scope of the local investigators because basic changes in the system were needed requiring centralized decision-making. Another drawback of the operations research was the concentration on one small aspect of the system, the one perceived by the investigators as the single limiting factor in a highly complex system. Improvement in this one aspect did not necessarily enhance the productivity or functioning of the whole system, as frequently more than one problem existed. More responsive and timely research methods are needed if operations research results are to affect decision-making.

Research methodologies are needed which permit researchers to objectively and systematically understand the many factors affecting the success of PHC strategies reliant upon CHW. Analytical tools must be developed to enable researchers to measure more precisely the inputs, operational processes, outputs, effects, and even impacts of CHW service delivery activities. These tools are based upon carefully planned management information systems that indicate process inputs and outputs as coverage; health worker training, knowledge and compliance; patient compliance; and screening or diagnostic accuracy. Operations research has been used widely in family planning, but to a much smaller extent in health programs (Gallen and Rineheart, 1986).

Operations research functions to identify problems, analyze the situation, and suggest solutions. Yet further efforts to develop techniques and tools for more responsive and rapid systems analysis and subsequent training in these methods could greatly enhance the functioning of both primary health care and other related systems

The results of basic and epidemiologic research appear to have a greater likelihood of rapid, broad applicability compared to operations and social science research. These frequently are bound to the cultural, societal, political, and system context and may take years to gradually change.

Present Status of Biomedical Research

The new biotechnology research techniques offer a historic opportunity for rapid discovery of new tools for prevention, diagnosis, epidemiological surveillance, and treatment of the endemic diseases of the tropics. A remarkable number of new vaccines, drugs, and diagnostic techniques will be available within ten years for preventing infectious diseases and also for simplifying family planning. Those predicted by the United States Institute of Medicine (IOM) to be licensed within five years are listed in Table 12 and those predicted for licensure within ten years are listed in Table 13 (Hatcher, *et al.*, 1986; IOM, 1984 and 1986; Spieler, 1985). The fulfillment of these predictions depends on research efforts continuing at the present level plus prompt completion of field studies. Clinical trials may be the greatest hurdle before any of these new vaccines, drugs, and diagnostic tools may be utilized. They require large, carefully followed populations and experienced field study teams, and sometimes must occur in poorly accessible areas.

Table 12.   New Vaccines Licenced Within Five Years

Bordetella pertussis	— Acellular
Hemophilus influenza Type B	— Conjugated polysaccharide
Hepatitis A	— Attenuated live virus or subunit vaccine
Herpes simplex 1 and 2	— Glycoprotein
Influenza virus A and B	— Purified hemagglutinin/ neuraminidase proteins
	— Attenuated live virus
Neisseria meningitidis	— Conjugated polysaccharide
Parainfluenza virus	— Subunit
Rabies virus	— Vero cell
	— Glycoprotein
	— Attenuated live virus
Respiratory syncytial virus	— Glycoprotein
	— Attenuated live virus
Rotavirus	— Attenuated live virus
Salmonella typhi	— Ty21a strain
Streptococcus pneumoniae	— Conjugated polysaccharide
Vibrio Cholera	— Purified antigen

Table 13.   New Vaccines Licensed Within Ten Years

Dengue	— Attenuated live virus
E. Coli	— Enterotoxigenic
Human immunodeficiency virus	
Japanese B encephalitis	
Mycobacterium leprae	
Neisseria gonorrhoeae	
Plasmodium spp.	
Salmonella typhi	— Aromatic amino acid dependent strain
Streptococcus Group A	
Streptococcus Group B	
Vibrio cholera	— Attenuated live bacteria
Antipregnancy vaccine	— Human chorionic gonadotropin beta subunit
	— Ovine luteinizing hormone
Male antifertility vaccine	

Vaccines

The ideal vaccine for the developing world should include the following characteristics: (1) It should be a single-dose agent that induces life-long or at least long-lasting immunity. (2) The immunity induced should prevent carriage and transmission of infection in addition to the disease (herd immunity). (3) It should remain stable at tropical temperatures for long periods; and (4) it should involve easy administration through an inexpensive disposable device or vehicle not requiring sterilization between use (unlike most needles and syringes), preferably administered by a primary health worker. (5) It should be inexpensive (ideally much less than one dollar per dose, and (6) efficacious at birth or shortly thereafter. (7) It should have minimal side effects, and (8) be safely used in combination with other immunogens for simultaneous administration. (9) Immunity should be induced shortly after administration (effective in outbreak control). (10) Population screening for vaccine acceptance should be easy (*e.g.*, the smallpox vaccine by skin scarification leaves a visible scar verifiable by a field worker); and (11) it should be of high purity so that the potential for cross-reactivity is very small.

None of the presently available vaccines possesses all of these characteristics and many in the process of development fall short of this ideal. One of the most prominent candidates, incorporating many of these attributes, is a viral carrier vaccine using vaccinia or another related virus which can integrate the genetic determinants of many proteins into its DNA and simultaneously immunize against a variety of antigens (see below).

• *Biomedical Techniques.* Among the approaches for new vaccine development are the following (Channock, 1985; IOM, 1984 and 1986; Lerner, *et al.*, 1985):

1. Purified viral proteins. The currently available plasma-derived Hepatitis B surface antigen and influenza virus subunit vaccines use the purified viral protein approach. The immunogenic proteins are purified from a mixture containing the dead virus. This method probably will be supplanted by the newer biomedical techniques.

2. Proteins from recombinant DNA. The genetic material responsible for production of the immunity-inducing antigen is incorporated into the genome of another bacteria, yeast, or animal cell. The cell or organism replicates and produces the protein,

ideally in large quantities. The protein then requires purification before administration. An example of this technique is the new recombinant Hepatitis B vaccine, in which the DNA sequence coding for the surface antigen is incorporated into yeast and activated to synthesize the protein. The major advantage of animal cells in this system is their close biochemical proximity to human cells, the targets for the pathogens. This metabolic similarity is important for the production of some protein immunogens (*e.g.,* the major Human Immunodeficiency Virus (HIV) surface protein) as they require glycosylation in order to function as immunogens, and animal cells have the ability to glycosylate the proteins appropriately.

3. *Genetic variants.* This approach results in attenuated mutants similar to the presently available poliomyelitis, measles, mumps, and rubella vaccines. These older vaccines have the potential for reversion to virulent forms, but through the use of the new genetic engineering techniques, mutant strains incapable of reversion can be developed. Several methods have been tried: introduction of a lethal mutation, for example, into the DNA polymerase so the virus can enter the cell but cannot replicate; deletion of a specific gene needed for virulence; and gene reassortment, or segregation of the genes responsible for protection from those responsible for disease so that the virus retains its infectiousness and immunogenicity without its virulence. This approach has primarily been applied to viruses but is potentially useful for bacteria. One of the new typhoid variants is missing the epimerase gene so that multiplication is limited.

4. *Synthetic polypeptides.* The amino acid sequence of a specific antigenic viral, bacterial, or other microorganism polypeptide can be defined and then chemically synthesized. These peptides may be so small that they will not elicit an immune response when administered alone but will require mixing with an adjuvant or bonding to larger molecules to induce immunity. These synthetic antigens can be expected to have fewer side effects because of their purity. Moreover, they cost relatively little when produced on a large scale. A peptide vaccine based on specific sequences in the Hepatitis B surface antigen under development is an example.

5. *Recombinant viruses and bacteria.* The gene for a protective protein is incorporated into the genome of a carrier virus or bacteria

that produces a relatively benign infection in man. When the organism infects, the immunity to this protein is induced. The vaccinia virus (smallpox vaccine) has been studied most thoroughly, but adenovirus, herpes virus, and BCG remain possibilities. Vaccinia recombinants have induced significant immunity to hepatitis B surface antigen, rabies, herpes simplex and influenza in animals. They have an enormous potential for carrying many genes and simultaneously immunizing for several different diseases because at least 22 kb of exogenous DNA can be inserted into vaccinia virus without diminishing its infectivity for cell culture. BCG is a safe and widely used vaccine, having been administered to over a billion and a half persons (Godal, 1987). It induces strong T cell responses and its genome should prove to be a useful vector for genes coding for protective antigens against a variety of diseases endemic in the developing countries. This possibility is being explored in studies currently being sponsored by the NIH, The Rockefeller Foundation, and the WHO Programme for Tropical Disease Research.

6. *Anti-Idiotype Antibodies.* The idiotype of an antibody is located at or near the antigen combining site. Antibodies directed against the idiotype may mimic the three-dimensional conformation of the antigen. Anti-idiotypic antibodies directed against HBsAg and retrovirus capsid proteins induce immunity in animals to infection by these organisms. Anti-idiotypic antibodies produce immunity without the administration of any components of a pathogen, thereby averting the possibility of disease from the vaccine.

• *Needs and Constraints.* Research is in progress for many vaccines potentially of great health benefit for the developing world using the techniques listed above. Nevertheless, many severe diseases are remarkable in their absence from Tables 1 and 2. The vaccine for tuberculosis, BCG, appears efficacious only in limited circumstances despite more than sixty years of use and study. Because of the enormous burden of illness from the Mycobacterium, greater priority should be placed on research for this disease. Several of the respiratory pathogens have little prospect for vaccines in the near future, notably *Staphylococcus aureus, Mycoplasma pneumoniae,* and the common cold. Diverse diarrheal diseases lack adequate vaccines, *e.g.,* the Shiga bacillus, enteropathogenic *E. coli,* and Campylobacter. Many of the parasitic illnesses: amebiasis, hookworm, trypanosomiasis, onchocerciasis, ascariasis, and leishmaniasis, are undergoing intensive study although prospects for vaccines in the next decade are dismal. The importance of sexually transmitted diseases is increasingly recognized, particularly in Africa where rapid socio-economic shifts have disrupted traditional societies and culture, resulting in greater transmission. Syphilis, gonorrhoea, chlamydia, and AIDS all have poor prospects for the short-term development of efficacious, inexpensive vaccines.

Biomedical technology has enormously improved the prospects for development of beneficial vaccines, using a variety of techniques: anti-idiotypic antibodies, polypeptide synthesis, purified proteins, recombinant proteins, genetic variants, and recombinant viruses. Nevertheless, considerable concentrated effort and resources are required to reap the potential fruits of the biotechnology revolution. The current status of vaccine research, the need and constraints for large-scale field trials, and particularly neglected infections should be considered when judging priorities for future research efforts.

In spite of the exciting prospects for disease control suggested by these new vaccines, the history of health services in the tropics demonstrates that a new and effective tool does not necessarily ensure that the disease in question will be controlled. Not only should new tools be free of side effects, low cost, mass-applicable and simple in operation, but also there must be an appropriate strategy for delivery to the target population. The endeavor of disease control must involve the entire voyage of the vaccine or drug from the factory to the village.

Diagnostic and Surveillance Tools

Improved diagnostic tools will foster both patient care and public health. For patient care, enhanced diagnostic capability will promote more specific and successful treatment of illnesses that can be caused by a variety of infecting agents, such as pneumonia, fever, liver enlargement, bloody diarrhea, and swollen glands. Simple tests for the causal organism will ensure accurate, rapid diagnosis and hasten initiation of efficacious treatment. For public health, these tools will aid in: (1) monitoring and surveillance, (2) assessment of disease control efforts, and (3) planning through the provision of the epidemiologic data required to quantify incidence and prevalence. Examples of potential applications outside of infectious disease diagnosis include identification of drug resistance in microorganisms and insects, rapid assessment of oral rehydration solution concentration, measurement of hemoglobin levels, testing of water supplies and environment for toxins or pathogens, identification of cancers and neoplasia, and detection of carriers of typhoid (Caskey, 1987). Improved diagnostics will also benefit family planning acceptance. For example, better ovulation-detection methods for the fertile period should make the periodic abstinence method more reliable and acceptable.

The desirable features sought for diagnostics for the developing world include: simplicity of use, adaptability to local conditions, stability, minimal need for instrumentation, lowest possible cost, speed, and accuracy. For patient care, the individual test should ideally take less than an hour and be read in a minimally furnished community clinic or even in the home of the community health worker; for epidemiologic surveys, a slower test adapted for batch processing is satisfactory. Types of vehicles under development include: slide agglutinations, filter paper blots, dipsticks, capillary tubes, small test tubes, and plastic envelopes.

The examination of clinical specimens always carries several inherent difficulties: care must be taken in obtaining the specimen to ensure that the appropriate source is sampled and that the specimen is of good quality. The stage of the illness may affect the results, and the health worker must be protected from infections transmitted by body fluids. For example, sputum may be heavily contaminated with saliva, organisms may be present intermittently or be carried asymptomatically and not cause the present illness, use of blood carries the risk of spread of hepatitis B or possibly HIV. Many specimens may require pretreatment prior to testing to concentrate the pathogen or antigen or release it from an intracellular site. Urine is the easiest source to work with as it is readily obtainable except from young infants, and the kidney concentrates many antigens.

• *Techniques.* Diagnostic methods under development may be divided under two headings (Proceedings, 1986c): *Immunoassay* and *Nucleic Acid Hybridization*. Immunoassay involves the mechanism of antibodies combining with specific antigens. The antigen may derive from a microorganism causing an infection or it can be a toxin, vitamin, chemical, or other compound. In the past, the test has employed polyclonal antibodies directed against a variety of antigens associated with an organism. However, the use of monoclonal antibodies has markedly improved the sensitivity and specificity of the assays. The immunoassay techniques include: (1) ELISA (Enzyme Linked Immunoadsorbant Assay). This assay can be read visually for a qualitative or semiquantitative result. It can be performed individually or in batches, and the reagents are stable. But the present format generally requires a substantial time commitment from a skilled technologist, and the reagents are quite expensive to produce. (2) *Immunofluorescence.* This assay requires the use of a properly maintained fluorescence microscope and a skilled microscopist. (3) *Agglutination assays.* These are inexpensive, simple, visually readable and stable procedures, but lack adequate sensitivity unless the antigen is preconcentrated.

In *nucleic acid hybridization assays,* the DNA or RNA of the "probe" combines with identical complementary nucleic acid fragments in the specimen under examination. These probes can identify any living organism, be it virus, bacterium, or cellular parasite, by a certain stretch of nucleic acid that belongs exclusively to that organism. Thus, probes may be developed for nucleic acids that are exclusive to one species of bacterium or viral strain or common to all species in a genus or class of protozoa, for example.

The develpment and use of these probes can be described simply. Once a nucleic acid sequence that is unique to a particular pathogen has been identified, recombinant gene methods are employed to produce hundreds of copies of the sequence for use as probes. The probes are then radiolabeled or tagged with easily identified molecules, like biotin or enzymes, and denatured into single-stranded versions. The specimen, whether blood, urine, feces, penile exudate, or vaginal smear, is usually handled in one of two ways—in solution or as a solid fixed on a filter or other appropriate holder. The probe, when added to either the solution or the prepared filter, will hybridize with the complementary DNA or RNA sequence wherever it is present, and then the excess is removed. The solution or filter is then analyzed for the presence of labeled probe. If the label is present, the specimen is positive for the organism. If it is not, the specimen is negative (Merz, 1987).

The nucleic acid hybridization assays are less well developed than the immunoassays but the potential for future use is much greater. It has the following advantages: Its specificity can be engineered depending on the amount of homology and number of base pairs involved. (The sensitivity may be low when DNA is used as the target since there may be only one copy per cell, but use of RNA which has multiple copies may improve sensitivity). The reagents are stable and relatively inexpensive: Multiple analyses are possible on the same specimen, and nonspecific cross-reactivity is much less than with immunoassays and unaffected by surface modifications in the organism.

• *Current Status.* Few diagnostic and surveillance tools are presently available for use in the primary health care or community setting in the developing world. Group A Streptococcal and *Chlamydia trachomatis* immunoassays are used in physicians' offices, but would require modification before they could be cost-effectively applied to field use in developing countries. Nucleic acid probes have been developed for a variety of infectious agents, including enterotoxigenic *E. coli*, *Neisseria gonorrhoea*, *Leishmania mexicana*, *Plasmodium falciparum* and *P. vivax*, Salmonella spp., Shigella spp., cytomegalovirus, adenovirus, hepatitis B virus, and the enteroviruses. While some of these probes are still restricted to experimental use, others are commercially available in kits (Merz, 1987; Proceedings, 1986a, 1986b, 1986c; Wirth, *et al.*, 1986). Many others have been developed in the laboratory but lack adequate field testing to determine sensitivity and specificity and will require simplification and a decrease in cost before they are ready for widespread use in the developing world. Amebiasis, giardiasis, typhoid, Group B streptococcus, among others, represent examples at this stage of development. At present, the malaria DNA-hybridization test appears as sensitive as good microscopy and ovulation-detection methods for use in family planning are rapidly advancing (Wirth, *et al.*, 1986). However, these still require simplification before widespread field use is possible. It is unclear if any others will be available within five years.

Nucleic acid probes will assume a prominent role particularly in the diagnosis of organisms that are expensive, difficult, and slow to culture in the laboratory or to identify by other means. Tuberculosis, *Campylobacter*, *Mycoplasma*, *Legionella*, influenza virus, cytomegalovirus, the hepatitis viruses, and picornaviruses (which have a common structure but great antigenic diversity and are thus able to elude antibody assays) are good examples of this category. Recognition of resistance genes in bacteria, viruses, protozoa, insects, and other vectors will be another important use of this technique (Merz, 1987; Proceedings, 1986a, 1986b, 1986c; Caskey, 1987).

An enormous potential exists for improving both patient care and public health services through future developments in diagnostic and information management tools. Although the use of nucleic acid probes is still in its infancy, they seem destined to transform the diagnosis of infectious disease and public health surveillance. Few, if any, diagnostic tools will be ready for field use within five years, however, since more work is needed to decrease costs, simplify procedures, and perform field tests. Criteria for prioritizing research and development on diagnostic and information technologies might include: assessing the burden of disease caused by the infecting organism (toxin or nutrient deficiency), efficacy of therapeutic and/or control measures available, status of presently available diagnostic and surveillance tools, status of research and development and cost for developing better tools. Based on these criteria, several priority areas for patient care include tuberculosis, respiratory infections, amebiasis, typhoid, and malaria. For epidemiology and disease surveillance, priorities include malaria in mosquitoes, mosquito species, resistance in insects and malaria, water purity, toxins, and food quality and contamination.

Drugs

Through efforts spearheaded by the World Health Organization's Special Programme on Tropical Disease Research, several new drugs for tropical diseases have been developed. These include mefloquine for malaria (already licensed), ivermectin for filariasis, and difluoromethyl ornithine against African Trypanosomiasis. Praziquantal for schistosomiasis is ready to begin field trials for use in control programs. Several other chemical derivatives of the active component of the Chinese herb "Quinghaosu" are being developed, as agents effective against drug resistant malarial infections (Maurice and Pearce, 1987).

• *Needs and Constraints.* Newer compounds are needed based on the specific interruption of metabolic pathways unique to pathogenic organisms, which are efficacious either as a single dose or in multiple doses over a short period of time with little or no adverse reactions. They should be capable of easy incorporation into the primary health care system, and be introduced with a mechanism for monitoring and controling adverse reactions at a national level.

Breaking the dangerous partnership between malnutrition and infections, predominantly manifested as the Diarrhea-Pneumonia-Malnutrition complex, is achieved mainly through immunization and chemotherapy in the primary care setting complemented by measures to deal with malnutrition. Drugs and vaccines effective against major pathogens of this complex are in need of further development. The long lag period between discovery of a drug and its practical end use in the clinic, health center, and the field, together with the other issues connected with drugs for health development, are dealt with later in this section.

One of major constraints for rapid application of all the biomedical discoveries is the need for large clinical trials and the shortage of places in tropical countries in which to perform them. These require a carefully studied population and locale, epidemiologic expertise on site, and access to rapid analytic capability. Few developing country institutions and sites are capable of undertaking trials involving the many thousands of individuals usually needed. This stage of research and development is also one of the most expensive.

In order for the predicted new health technologies to actually come into use, continuing investment in biomedical research, at least at the current levels, is required. Increased funding can be expected to accelerate the pace of discovery. Priorities would be those conditions causing the greatest disease burden in which drugs and vaccines may not be available within the next decade. Complementary efforts to increase the capacity for field evaluation are required to ensure that these drugs and tools are rapidly utilized.

Research Priorities

The priorities for research comprise a number of levels and types. Many of the research topics can be grouped into related areas: for example, (based on Figure 3), (a) diseases and conditions, such as low birth weight, sexually transmitted diseases, respiratory infections, psychological and mental illness, malnutrition, etc., (b) the community level determinants, such as health services, safety, behavior promotion, water supply and sanitation, and (c) the societal or foundation level determinants, such as communication, education, environment. Research priorities can also be analyzed by (a) need for developing or delivering a control measure such as a vaccine or drugs, (b) by types of research (basic, applied, social, epidemiologic, health services and operations).

The following will describe research priorities by type of research. This method helps delineate the resources needed to carry out the investigations, since specific scientific skills, equipment, and locations are needed at each of the different levels of research: basic, epidemiologic, operations and health services, and social and intersectoral research.

Priorities for Basic Research

The new techniques of biotechnology open the door to unprecedented opportunities. The three priority areas for basic biomedical research based on the foregoing principles of burden of illness and interventions available are: vaccines, drugs, and diagnostic and surveillance tools. Of these three, vaccines are the most important health-fostering measure, since they prevent both morbidity and mortality from infection, and transmission to others. In contrast, drugs and diagnostic tools can help prevent mortality and severe morbidity, but usually, the patient must have some degree of ill health before seeking appropriate therapy from the health care system.

Other potential areas for great advances using these techniques are environmental sanitation and agriculture (crop improvement). Organisms that will detoxify and purify chemical waste, poisons, and sewage are already undergoing field trials. Potentially, these organisms may be used to remove hazardous chemicals from the environment, to purify water supplies, and to decontaminate and cleanse biological wastes. These hazards become a mounting problem with the population explosion, and increasing urbanization and industrialization of the globe. The future will find need for increased efficiency, multipurpose organisms, that are easy to use and inexpensive. Such research needs as described above will inevitably be addressed by the biotechnologic revolution.

The cost of research and development for vaccines, drugs, diagnostics, and environmental organisms across-the-board is fairly similar. Each area requires extensive field trials. Environmental organisms and diagnostics probably require less human testing for reactions and toxicity prior to licensing, which frequently is the most expensive phase. On the other hand, testing environmental organisms to assess their effect and possible disruption of the ecosystem represents new and possibly costly territory. The cost to prepare a vaccine for end use, as it stands now, totals $20 to $30 million.

• *Vaccines.* The Institute of Medicine analysis lists several vaccines as high priorities for research (IOM, 1984; 1984). In many cases, however, the delay to future availability may not be substantially shortened by increasing the funding, since many await only completion of the planned human trials. The time constraints for human trials is difficult to shorten because Phase I, II, III, and IV trials must be performed serially (See Table 11). Currently, few field areas in developing countries have the manpower and expertise to carry out the extensive population monitoring required. The lack of field sites has become a notable bottleneck for several TDR drug discoveries. A few diseases can be identified for which additional funding for vaccine development would likely substantially decrease the delay to field trials and subsequent licensing. These include the following:

1.   *Tuberculosis vaccine.*   The efficacy of the present BCG vaccine remains questionable despite almost six decades of use. Few labs are presently working on new vaccine formulations.

2.   *Respiratory vaccines.* Vaccines that are efficacious for long-term administration to newborns or young infants are particularly needed. The most important of these agents is the polysaccharide *Strep. pneumoniae. H. influenza* polysaccharide has now been attached to a protein adjuvant that appears to increase its immunogenicity in infants. Developments in vaccines for the respiratory viruses, such as influenza, parainfluenza, respiratory syncytial virus, and the common cold would be hastened by additional funding.

3.   *Group B Strep.* This organism was identified as a priority for research and development in the Institute of Medicine analysis for the United States, but was not considered in the developing country analysis because little epidemiologic evidence is available concerning its natural history in the developing nations. In the United States, this organism is the major pathogen in maternal postpartum sepsis and neonatal sepsis. It is a major cause of neonatal pneumonia, and evidence accumulates concerning its role in precipitating premature rupture of membranes and premature labor. Through these syndromes, Group B Strep is a major cause of maternal morbidity (and mortality if treatment is delayed as occurs in developing countries), neonatal mortality, and low birth weight. Several recent studies have documented its importance in many parts of the world (Walsh, in press). Currently, phase I human trials have been completed and it awaits funding before further tests can begin.

4. *Syphilis.*   Little recent research has occurred on this disease, despite its extensive burden of illness. The introduction of penicillin treatment for syphilis lulled many public health planners into believing that the threat had faded. Its importance, particularly in Africa where it contributes greatly to low birth weight and neonatal mortality, has only recently been recognized.

5. *Amebiasis vaccine.* Several prototype formulations are presently undergoing animal trials. Increased funding would increase the number of labs involved in the development and hasten the process of identification and formulation of the ideal immunogens and facilitate human trials.

6. *Immunoadjuvants and immunopotentiators for the purified antigens now being synthesized, with the goal of developing one-dose, long-lasting immunity.*   As described in the section on status of research, carrier organisms capable of integrating into their nucleic acids the genes coding for several protein immunogens and simultaneously conferring immunization to the host offer an enormous potential. A system which can immunize in one visit for multiple disease without the need of several boosters, would enhance coverage enormously. Vaccinia, adenovirus, herpes, and polio viruses have been studied in laboratory settings and vaccinia has undergone several animal trials. BCG, which has been safely administered to billions of persons, has an enormous genome potentially capable of carrying many additional gene codes.

7. *Increasing the temperature stability of present (and future) vaccines.*   This area borders on applied research. The need for a cold chain (refrigerated delivery) has complicated the delivery of vaccines to the periphery (field). The stability and ease of administration of the smallpox vaccine contributed to the successful eradication of smallpox, since vaccinators could easily carry a supply of the vaccine and bifurcated needles in their pockets as they rode bikes and oxcarts or walked through inaccessible rural areas. With a heat-stable vaccine, community health workers could maintain a supply and administer the vaccine locally as new infants reached the appropriate age.

8. *Vaccines for use in family planning for both men and women.* Antifertility vaccines to aid in child spacing will likely improve the outcome of pregnancy both for the mother and infant and improve the chances of successful growth and development for the child.

- *Drugs*   High priority drugs include:

1.   *Tuberculosis.*   In addition to vaccine development, an agent is needed for short duration chemotherapy. Lack of compliance with the 6 to 24 months' course of treatment needed for cure with the present vaccine inhibits successful control programs.

2.   *Antiviral agents.*   Agents for influenza, parainfluenza, herpes, AIDS, among others are needed. Drugs for the respiratory viruses must be inexpensive and safe enough to be used by village health workers. Treatment must start within a few hours of onset of symptoms. Otherwise they are likely to be ineffective.

3.   *Antihelminthics.*   A single drug is needed efficacious in a small number of doses against a broad spectrum of intestinal and tissue helminths.

- *Diagnosis and Surveillance*   Tools in diagnosis and surveillance for the diseases with the greatest burden of illness include: rapid assessment of oral rehydration solution concentration, measurement of hemoglobin levels, testing quality of water supplies, identification of malaria parasites in mosquitoes and for drug resistance, and identification of respiratory pathogens.

Applied Research

Applied research entails many different types of studies but generally implies efforts to improve existing technologies so that they can be used widely. These include techniques for manufacturing, distribution, or administration methodologies and development of better vaccines, therapeutics, and diagnostic tools. Examples include engineering improvements, such as development of a single-use, disposable combined needle and syringe, or better jet injectors for administering vaccines, and the development of low cost, low maintenance, technologically appropriate water pumps and latrines. Other examples utilizing biomedical techniques include improved temperature stable vaccines, immunoadjuvants, and development of vehicles such as BCG or vaccinia virus to induce immunity to many different diseases simultaneously (Lechat, 1986).

Usually a technological modification costs relatively little compared to the cost of conducting field trials. When a product requires many modifications, however, the resource investments can become expensive.

The priorities for applied research based on information presented in earlier sections and upon discussions with others in the field of international health are as follows:

1.   Efforts are needed to ease and simplify the provision of immunizations globally. The current immunizations are the most cost-effective health interventions available (see Table 9). Many others will shortly become available. The new immunizations can be distributed using the channels now established. These efforts include:

    a.   Improved heat stabilization of vaccines so that the cold chain apparatus and procedures are not needed.

    b.   Improved administration equipment. This combined with heat stable vaccines will allow long-term storage and availability of vaccines in the community or clinic so that either village health workers or even community leaders could ensure immunization of the appropriate target groups. Vaccines could be carried easily by health workers on foot or on bicycles visiting homes and communities. These technologies would help ensure thorough immunization coverage.

    c.   Development of less expensive, technologically simplified manufacturing processes for vaccines and some drugs so that the developing world can become self-reliant by producing vaccines and drugs locally. A note of caution, the difficulties in production and quality control should not be underestimated. The UNDP/WHO program for setting up local quality control testing of imported supplies has had to overcome significant obstacles.

    d.   Development of immunogens and immunoadjuvant systems effective at birth or shortly after with one or a small number of doses.

    e.   Development of systems for the simultaneous administration of multiple immunogens; for example, chemically synthesized antigens combined with an adjuvant or carrier microorganism, such as BCG, or a virus with the nucleic acid of the antigen genes integrated within them.

2.   Development and dissemination of robust, inexpensive sanitary excreta disposal systems and water pumps. The technological development stage may be completed, but dissemination including local manufacture and quality control remain stumbling blocks.

Manufacture of low-cost, new-generation hand pumps has begun in several countries but expansion of this capacity is necessary. In addition, availability without correct use and maintenance results in minimal health benefit. Thus the educational component remains a cogent issue.

3.   Development of efficient health information systems to ease recording, reporting, compiling, and feedback of pertinent health information. These systems are invaluable for management, administration, problem-solving, and planning health care systems and should include process and impact measurements.

4.   Development, testing, and cost-effectiveness analysis of communication methods for health promotion. Films, radio reports, posters, flannel board drawings, lectures, television spots, among others, have been used for health education and promotion frequently without evaluation of effectiveness and analysis of costs. The applied research needs are for the development of effective tools for use in health promotion, and the related epidemiologic and economic research needs are the analysis of health impact. Communication can have an enormous impact but its role and ideal use has yet to be defined.

Epidemiological Research

Epidemiological research involves many types of studies; for example, examination of the natural history of disease; determination of the burden of illness; risk factor studies for low birth weight; burns and falls; impact of vitamin A deficiency; transmission patterns for infections, and clinical trials of interventions. This is an exceedingly important research area for many reasons, including the urgent need for such information in health planning and evaluation, and in identification of risk factors for delineating future health promotion strategies. The epidemiologic studies and clinical trials of interventions are the rate-limiting step before the population-based application of new interventions can commence.

1.   The primary constraint in this area is the need to identify populations suitable for large-scale field trials of interventions. The populations must be carefully censused, followed, and analyzed. The mortality and morbidity experience of its people and the endemicity, incidence, and prevalence of the various diseases must also be known. Community support must be established, and a cadre

of interested, trained investigators must be present on site together with a network of individuals trained in related fields, such as biostatistics, health, and social sciences. Along with institutional support, these factors must all be present to ensure the successful outcome of the studies. Several locations in the world are already conducting excellent field epidemiologic studies and can function as models for establishing others. Some examples include the International Center for Diarrheal Disease Research in Bangladesh; The British Medical Research Laboratory in the Gambia, the respiratory disease and malaria field sites in the highlands and coast of Papua, New Guinea; The Kasongo Primary Health Care Project in Zaire, among others. Other locations could become fine sites with some additional support for training, institutional strengthening, or enhanced efforts for population analysis. The numbers of trained scientists and strong research institutions has markedly increased in the last several decades, and many developing countries are presently able to train most of their own scientists locally, but the need for continuing support for training and institution strengthening remains.

Several interventions that await large-scale field trials since they have demonstrated efficacy in pilot studies include ivermectin for filariasis; new antimalarials; and difluoromethyl ornithine against African trypanosomiasis; treatment of acute respiratory infections under differing conditions and using different diagnostic algorithms and antibiotics; modified cooking stoves to improve efficient use of wood or other energy sources in order to decrease indoor air pollution, to decrease complicated respiratory infections, and to reduce the risk of infant and childhood household burns; bed nets for vector-transmitted infections; and others.

Other priorities for epidemiologic research include:

2.   Clinical trials of new drugs, vaccines, and diagnostic and surveillance tools, as mentioned above in regard to basic research needs.

3.   Investigation of the incidence, risk factors, and identification of potential interventions for injuries. Potential preventive and therapeutic interventions include low cost, technologically appropriate improvements in environmental safety, specific behaviors associated with high risk and possible methods for change. A historical review of the experience with injuries in several developed countries would complement the epidemiologic studies and may

rapidly provide leads for possible interventions. For example, the incidence of non-violent injuries in the United States appears to have declined in the last fifty years. Can any specific societal, environmental, or behavioral modifications account for this?

4. Infections in pregnancy as risk factors for low birth weight. Infections are associated with preterm delivery and excess pregnancy loss. Several of the most common organisms include Group B Strep, mycoplasmas, chlamydia (first exposure during pregnancy), and syphilis. Since low birth weight is so prevalent in many countries and carries with it such dire consequences, efforts to define risk factors and areas for interventions are key. Infections can be easily treated or vaccinations developed, while causes of low birth weight, such as anatomical deficiencies, require different and more extensive health strategies. These studies would also provide additional evidence for the importance of low birth weight so that more public health attention would be accorded to it.

5. Immunization of women to prevent pneumonia in their babies. Pneumonia is one of the most important causes of death in infants. Immunization would provide maternal antibody which would be transferred via placenta to the infant, affording protection during the first six months of life. In addition, immunization of the mother in some preliminary studies appears to prime the infant's immune system to better respond to this same immunogen at an earlier age.

6. Causes of mortality and morbidity and geographic differences, particularly among youth and young adults, the most socioeconomically productive members of society. These studies should begin with accumulation of information from a number of the populations presently under study in which the results have not yet been published. Investigations of this topic should complement the first epidemiologic research priority, namely, the identification of populations for future studies.

7. To lessen the burden of maternal mortality most efficiently, a better scientific basis is needed for deciding among the intervention strategies. The research needs entail, identification of risk factors, testing efficacy, sensitivity and specificity of systems for identification of high-risk pregnancies, and analysis of relative cost. The research can go on simultaneously with pilot projects based on the presently available information.

8.   Evaluation of the present EPI and CDD programs in terms of health impact. Efforts are under way, but actual demonstration of improved infant and child survival secondary to these efforts continues to elude program managers. Within the context of setting health priorities, the health impact of selective primary health care strategies has also yet to be confirmed, even though much foreign health aid is based on this idea. The lack of confirmation appears more related to the expense, time, effort, and ethics involved in setting up a controlled trial.

A topic presently under investigation that could lead to one of the most cost-effective interventions for averting childhood deaths is vitamin A supplementation. At least three large-scale field trials are presently under way and others will begin shortly.

Operational Research

Operational research involves the whole range of health services research and systems analysis, such as development and testing of surveillance, monitoring, and evaluation schemes. It is closely related and integrated into good management and administration schemes both for health services and for other intersectoral efforts for health promotion. It usually involves identification of constraints within a system, analysis of approaches and possible solutions, testing of the proposed solution in a pilot situation, and finally, implementing the solution widely while monitoring its success.

The need for operations research is obvious as health systems in many parts of the world have frequently had less of an impact than expected (APHA, 1982; Berman, *et al.*, 1986; Chen, 1986). Some of the components of health services needing research for improved effectiveness include: financing, health education and promotion, logistics and supply, training, supervision, management and administration, planning, community involvement, and political will. In addition to health systems, other health-related areas make use of operations research, such as implementing water and sanitation systems, communication, environmental change, and vector control, among others.

The costs of operations research in individual projects may be fairly small ($10-100,000 range). However, generalizability of findings, probability of improving the situation or system under study, and time-frame needed to generate results are some of the factors to consider when deciding on priorities.

The priorities for operations research are:

1.   The primary constraints upon strengthening existing health services appears to be the lack of adequate information about the functioning of the system at each level. A rapid, easy-to-use, efficient management information system would enhance responsiveness and administration. It would provide indicators or tools for use in analyzing a system, detecting problems, and receiving feedback about the results of modifications in the system. Using the current method, it could take months to years to identify and address problems that, when resolved, may not have as much impact as other less obvious problems.

Several programs are developing rapid epidemiologic assessment and diagnostic tools, namely PATH (DIATech), the U.S. National Academy of Sciences, and the Tropical Health and Evaluation units in Antwerp and London.

The Strengthening Health Services section of the WHO may be the appropriate venue (a) to coordinate the efforts of groups already addressing this issue, (b) to review status to stimulate further efforts, and (c) to test results through its field projects.

2.   Health services research. Despite the provisos mentioned above, health services research must be supported. Some of the components needing research for improved effectiveness include: health care financing (de Ferranti, 1983; World Bank, 1987b), health education and promotion, logistics and supply, training, supervision, management and administration, planning, community involvement, and political will. In addition to its potential for improving the health impact in a specific location, such research will serve to train experienced public health administrators.

3.   Improvement of surveillance systems through the identification of the minimal statistical information needed for assessment and evaluating methods for recording, reporting, and utilizing data.

4.   Improving appropriate community and individual use of water, sanitation facilities, and hygiene.

Social and Intersectoral Research

Social research covers anthropologic and intersectoral investigations, such as behavior, and the economic components of health promoting practices. Some examples of this type of research include: the identification of maternal or household practices that correlate with varying risks for infant and childhood diarrhea; determinants of choice of healthworker or healer used; correlates of compliance; economic costs of illness; cognitive psychology and sociology; impact of education, agriculture, and food supply on health; and family planning.

Since many intersectoral factors determine health as illustrated in Figure 3, research in this area may potentially have a marked impact on health. As in operations research, many of the topics covered in this field may be culturally or location specific and have relatively low generalizability. Moreover, studies must be selected carefully as the likelihood of success may be low. The priorities in this area include:

1.   Cost-effectiveness studies to assist policy and program decisions. Knowledge of the health impact of a variety of intersectoral efforts would support combined ventures in say vector control or environmental management, education, housing. The important topics for cost-effectiveness analysis include:

a.   Different types of health education (television, radio, home visits, clinic materials and discussions, women's groups).

b.   Primary education, particularly if it disaggregates curriculum content versus peer pressure versus attitudinal change resulting from schooling, making individuals more susceptible to future health education efforts, and disaggregating the components of the behavior change and the resulting changes in morbidity and mortality. Finally, measuring the effect of older sibling education on younger children.

c.   New types of housing and modification of old housing. Housing influences health determinants such as indoor pollution and respiratory infections, vector-borne disease transmission, such as Chagas Disease, injury risks, and personal hygiene to list only a few.

d.   Use of communication methods for health promotion and training, e.g., television, radio, and computer video (A system using videotapes and computer technology, permitting the trainee to view and interact directly with materials, at her own pace, without need for literacy. The system remarkably increases the speed and retention of learning.)

e.   Development, testing, and wide dissemination of simplified tools for cost-effectiveness analysis so that it may be used more widely. Analysis can thus occur in a timely fashion and aid decision-making.

2.   Education and its impact on health as discussed above under cost-effectiveness.

3.   Communication for health promotion. Analysis of areas in which it is most valuable and useful, how sustainable are its effects on behavior? What is the best way to reach those at highest risk?

4.   Development of methods for increasing community involvement, community and political commitment and will at various levels (national, regional, district, and local).

5.   Development of methods for improving equity in health; for reaching those at highest risk, the underserved, and those most vulnerable since these groups will have the poorest health.

Conclusions

From this lengthy list of priorities for different types of research, funding agencies must take into account the prospects for institutionalization of research, funding mechanisms, goals and strengths of the organization, among other regards. Priority does not imply exclusivity, because flexibility should be retained and some duplication of research efforts is desirable to insure successful outcome.

Most of the areas listed above are already under investigation. The following list represents those areas from the list above which have received limited investigation, yet it would appear would directly benefit health if they were to receive funding.

A program to increase research in any of these areas must include strengthening of institutions in the third world, linkages among scientists with common involvement, training, and capacity building, in addition to funding of actual investigations. These areas entail a range of research levels (basic, applied, epidemiologic, social) in order to assure rapid implementation of the results where they are needed most in the village. All of these topics are equally important and the listing does not imply ranking.

•   *Application of the powerful biotechnology techniques* to develop new, improved vaccines, drugs, diagnostics, and vector control techniques for those diseases with the highest morbidity and mortality.

•   *Identifying large field sites* for epidemiologic studies and field trials of vaccines, drugs, diagnostics, and other interventions. This includes census and mapping of the population, preliminary assessment of risk factors, and capacity building among institutions and individuals locally.

93

- *Innovation and examination of the role of communications* and the news media in health promotion and training (radio, television, video, computer video, etc.).

- *Operations and health services research* particularly capacity building and stimulating a problem-solving attitude or mode among all health workers.

- *Improving the efficiency and functioning of management information systems* so that they serve the health system practically. Innovation and evaluation of information systems may be considered part of operations research; however, it plays such a paramount role that it requires specific stress.

- *Tuberculosis* prevention and treatment through better vaccines and treatment.

- *Injuries.* Epidemiologic studies followed by development and testing of interventions.

- *Low Birth Weight.* Epidemiologic studies, development of interventions, and then evaluation and application. These should particularly include the study of maternal infection in pregnancy and its effect on the outcome of pregnancy for both the mother and infant. The cohort of mothers at high risk of maternal morbidity practically coincides with those at high risk of having low birth weight infants; therefore, studies in this area will benefit both mother and infants.

- *Acute respiratory infection.* Better preventive measures such as vaccines, prophylaxis, enviromental modification, increased breast-feeding; better therapeutic case management with better diagnostic agents and drug treatment; health services, operations, behavioral, and education innovation and study to improve effectiveness.

4 *Funding*

Health Services

Governmental and Nongovernmental Expenditures

Governments in developing countries spend between 1% and 22% of central expenditures on health. The average expenditure is approximately 3% for the poorest countries, increasing to 4-5% among the middle income countries (World Bank, 1987a). In addition, nongovernmental expenditures amount to an additional 20% to 400% (World Bank, 1987b). For example, in Burundi in 1982, public expenditures amounted to $3.52 per capita, while nongovernmental sources provided an additional $0.71. In contrast, in Uganda in 1982, public expenditures amounted to $1.91 while nongovernmental sources provided $9.73 (World Bank, 1987b).

The World Bank further estimates that 70% to 85% of the total expenditures on health are spent on curative services. These are used to treat and care for patients through health facilities and independent providers, and medicines. In contrast, only 10% to 20% goes to preventive services such as maternal and child health care (for example, immunization, growth monitoring, family planning, and promotion of better breast-feeding and weaning practices). Even less, 5% to 10%, goes to community services such as vector control programs, educational and promotional programs on health, and hygiene and monitoring of disease patterns (World Bank, 1987a,b). Preventive and community services exert the greatest influence on health for each dollar invested, but only a small share of expenditures are devoted to these. The cost effectiveness of some interventions is discussed later in this chapter.

Bilateral and Multilateral Aid

Many of the industrialized countries provide substantial sums annually to developing countries for health as shown in Table 14, from the Development Assistance Committee (DAC) of the Organization for Economic Cooperation and Development (OECD). This lists commitments for health aid from 1980 to 1985 from the developed countries of the world. The total in 1985 for the 14 member countries was $1,386.2 million. Other countries also provide health aid, such as Holland, the Soviet Union, and East Germany. This total includes training, institution building, primary health care development, and many other programs, and usually a small percentage funds health research.

Several multilateral agencies provide assistance in health, including WHO, UNICEF, UNDP, and the World Bank and regional banks, such as the African Development Bank. Since 1981, the World Bank has gradually increased its loans in the population, health, and nutrition arena. Projects approved in 1985 committed $148 million (World Bank, 1985). One of the regional banks, the African Development Bank, has provided loans averaging about $25 million annually for the past ten years.

UNICEF provides assistance for child health and development in developing countries totalling approximately $475 million annually.

The World Health Organization's budget for 1986-1987 was $543 million for the headquarters and regional programs in the industrialized and developing countries. It is very difficult to disaggregate funding for health in the developing world. Funding for the special programs for research is considered below (World Health Organization, 1986g).

Several large private voluntary organizations fund health, population, nutrition, and rural development including CARE, Save the Children, USA for AFRICA, World Vision, the World Council of Churches, and many other smaller church-related and private organizations. Estimating the total for health services would require disaggregating health and water and sanitation expenditures from those spent on intersectoral and other health-related or health-beneficial programs such as education or population or nutrition.

Table 14. Official Bilateral Commitments for Health Aid DAC Members, 1980-1985, $m

Country	1980	1981	1982	1983	1984	1985
Australia	4.4	1.9	3.6	10.6	13.6	12.3
Austria	0.1	0.1	1.2	0.3	0.1	1.4
Belgium[1]	12.5	10.2	7.2	8.4	30.2	24.5
Canada	12.8	0.5	17.6	24.2	28.8	45.4
Denmark	29.2	28.8	10.7	8.8	17.6	24.7
Finland	2.7	3.7	9.2	3.2	12.1	21.0
France[2]	441.9	440.8	443.5	432.6	362.8	166.6
Germany	101.9	51.2	89.9	49.2	42.3	52.9
Ireland	—	—	—	—	—	1.6
Italy	3.9	13.5	37.9	54.0	51.1	81.1
Japan	90.1	192.3	137.9	129.1	138.8	161.9
Netherlands	62.3	60.6	53.2	42.6	27.2	38.3
New Zealand	4.7	2.6	0.7	1.0	1.0	0.7
Norway	14.2	31.0	24.6	11.7	29.2	34.8
Sweden	26.0	37.2	32.2	25.1	34.1	44.0
Switzerland	4.0	9.8	4.6	11.8	1.9	14.4
United Kingdom	26.7	20.1	18.1	23.7	27.5	31.7
United States	429.9	431.7	408.8	514.4	355.0	628.9
DAC Countries	1,267.3	1,336.0	1,300.9	1,350.7	1,173.3	1,386.2
E.E.C.[3]	6.6	19.8	31.0	18.9	20.3	10.9

Source: Development Assistance Committee/OECD

1. Disbursements
2. Includes health and social security transfers to overseas territories and departments with the exception of 1985.
3. European Economic Community.

Tropical Health Research

The WHO estimates that more than $20 per capita is invested by the developed countries annually for health-related research. In contrast, the developing countries collectively spend approximately $0.10 per capita. Only about 5% of the world's scientists work in the developing world, and even these individuals are subject to the pressures of "brain drain" (WHO, 1986g).

Several international, bilateral, and national agencies support research to improve health in the developing world. The large international agencies supporting research include the World Health Organization (WHO), the United Nations Development Programme (UNDP), and the World Bank. The WHO through its special programs—Tropical Disease Research (TDR), Diarrheal Disease Control (CDD), Human Reproduction Program (HRP), Acute Respiratory Infections (ARI), Vaccine Development and Basic and Applied Vaccinology, and the newly initiated Safe Motherhood and AIDS—is one of the largest distributors of funds for research. Its funds come from other international and bilateral agencies. The UNDP contributes both to the WHO special programs and other international laboratories such as the International Center for Diarrheal Disease Research, Bangladesh (ICDDR,B), and manages its own research programs, such as the highly successful joint UNDP/World Bank effort to develop a low-cost, low-maintenance, sturdy hand pump. The World Bank both contributes to the WHO and its special programs and provides small loans within certain of its health programs for the development of scientific resources and expertise in developing countries and for operational research.

Bilateral agencies such as the United States Agency for International Development (AID), and the German, Swiss, Canadian, and Scandinavian development aid agencies support health and development research efforts as a small proportion of their health budget. Table 14 (p. 97) presents the amounts committed by the member countries of the Development Assistance Committee (DAC). These probably represent the major bilateral donors, but commitments from the Eastern Block countries, such as the Union of Soviet Socialists Republics and East Germany are not tallied by this group. In 1983-1984, the USSR gave $2.6 billion for non-military foreign aid. The proportion for health is unknown. In the same year, the US total was $8.2 billion (Poats, 1985).

Bilateral agencies usually contribute directly to the WHO and its special programs, to the support of international laboratories (such as the ICDDR,B), and distribute their own research funds, as well as subcontracting funds to other organizations for managing research on particular topics. The Canadian International Development Research Centre (IDRC) accepts proposals from researchers in developing countries and manages its own program.

National Governments support health research, but usually a tiny proportion is spent on tropical health related issues. For example, out of the total budget of $2-3 billion for the United States National Institutes of Health (NIH), about $50 million is spent on diarrheal disease, acute respiratory infections, and the major parasitic diseases (Office of Technology Assessment, 1985). This amount does not include the funding for AIDS research, as it is not one of the traditional health problems of the tropics.

Pharmaceutical manufacturers around the world have invested in new drugs, vaccines, and diagnostic reagents for use in tropical diseases.

Each of these sources of funds will be considered separately.

MULTILATERAL AGENCIES

World Health Organization

The Tropical Disease Research Programme (TDR) budget for the biennium 1982-1983 comprised total obligations of approximately $50 million of which 25% was spent on research capability strengthening and 65% ($32.5 million) for research and development for the six diseases: malaria, schistosomiasis, leprosy, leishmaniasis, trypanosomiasis (African and Chagas), and filariasis. The budget for the biennium 1984-1985 was approximately the same, although the final tally is not available at this writing (TDR, 1987). Only a small proportion of these funds were invested in epidemiologic, social, and economic research and the vast majority of the money was spent for biomedical research, institution strengthening and training.

During the 1984-1985 biennium the CDD program received US $15.3 million, which was 25% more than that received during the previous biennium and about a third was spent on research. The three objectives of the program are: (A) to develop new or improved methods for prevention and treatment of diarrheal diseases caused by infection by supporting biomedical and epidemiological research; (B) to improve the performance of national CDD programs through operational research; (C) to enhance the capabilities of developing country institutions to conduct research on diarrheal diseases through institutional development activities. During the 1986-1987 biennium, the expected budget will total around US$ 19 million with US$ 7 million for research activities involving immunology, microbiology, and vaccine development; case management; and epidemiology and disease prevention (WHO, 1986f).

During the 1984-1985 biennium, the ARI program totaled $1.8 million and 60% came from the regular WHO budget. In the 1986-1987 biennium, the program will expand to $2.5 million and half will come from outside sources. The program involves three main components: health services, research, and promotion and information dissemination. The health services component first established the basic procedures for case management and now has moved into implementation and development of management and evaluation tools. Research has focused on the critical issues in case management, while promotion and information dissemination has included publication of a newsletter and establishing a network of involved individuals (WHO, 1986d). Current budget figures were not available for the communicable disease and vaccine program.

The Safe Motherhood program began in 1987 with a projected budget of $5 million for three years. Part of this budget will be spent on programs and part on primarily epidemiologic and operations research.

Other multilateral agencies

The United Nations Development Programme (UNDP), through its Division for Global and Interregional Programmes, funds research that will benefit health throughout the developing world. Its funds are primarily expended through commitments to other international organizations, such as WHO and its special programs mentioned above, in addition to Strengthening Health Services, vaccine quality control in manufacturing, and the ICDDR,B. The joint UNDP/World Bank program for the development of low-cost, low-maintenance, sturdy, simple hand pump and sanitation devices has been highly successful. This program also focuses on effluent recycling schemes involving biogas, irrigation and fertilization with effluent, and fish ponds. Other programs deal with methods for enrolling women to encourage installation, use, and maintenance of water supplies and sanitation facilities as well as communication for health promotion.

NATIONAL GOVERNMENTS

United States

The Department of Defense (DOD), NIH, Centers for Disease Control (CDC), and AID expend the largest amounts on tropical disease research. The latest figures available date from 1983, when the DOD spent $14 million on biomedical research for the six TDR diseases, diarrheal disease, and arboviral infections; the National Institute of Allergy and Infectious Diseases of the NIH spent $48 million on diarrheal and enteric infection, ARI, and tropical diseases; CDC $5 million on TDR, diarrheal diseases and ARI; AID $14 million. The AID funds went to the ICDDR,B; malaria vaccine development, vector control efforts, diarrheal, ARI and tropical disease research (OTA, 1985). The total US government commitment for 1983 was approximately $81 million largely for biomedical research.

Since 1983, AID has made greater efforts to expand operational and applied research with special contracts for vaccine field trials, operational research on primary health care (PRICOR I and II), diarrheal disease (ADDR), health care financing, diagnostic methods (DIATECH which funds efforts to devise and test low cost, marketable diagnostic products from laboratory discoveries), and soon, maternal health. Nonetheless, all of these efforts have probably amounted to only $4-5 million annually. The figures for 1983 do not include expenditures on AIDS research, which has accelerated rapidly and now amounts to well over $100 million annually.

Other National Governments

As mentioned previously, developing countries invest very little on health-related research, and only 5% of working scientists live there. Mexico, Brazil, China, and India each have national research funding organizations and institutions. The smaller, poorer countries have practically no research capacity.

Each of the industrialized countries has a health research organization or funding body which concentrates on diseases of highest priority to its citizens and expends relatively little on problems of the developing world. The British Medical Research Council, and the German Max Planck Institutes are examples. Meager information could be uncovered that disaggregated investments made in tropical health research. No information could be found on health research investments by the Eastern Block countries.

PRIVATE FOUNDATIONS

Several private foundations in the United States and in the industrialized countries have funded tropical health-related research: *e.g.,* Clark, Sasakawa, Rockefeller, MacArthur, Wellcome. MacArthur has one of the largest monetary commitment with $4 million committed annually for 5 years beginning in 1983. These funds were earmarked to support centers of excellence to apply the techniques of modern biology to parasitic diseases. The Rockefeller Foundation's Health Sciences program totals approximately $10 million annually and has categories for Great Neglected Diseases (GND), Clinical Epidemiology, New Age of Vaccines, and Coping with Biomedical and Health Information. Both the GND and the Clinical Epidemiology components have established networks of scientists and strong collaborative bonds amongst groups in developed and developing countries. The foundation has usually provided only limited funds for each research unit (not exceeding $150,000 over several years) and the majority of research funding has come from other sources. The Clinical Epidemiology Network has rapidly expanded and now spends about $3 million annually. The Clark Foundation in the past funded schistosomiasis research, but more recently has become interested in preventable causes of blindness, such as trachoma. Wellcome Trust recently stopped its schistosomiasis research program in preference to studying the antecedents and risk factors for hypertension among urban slum dwellers in Nairobi.

PHARMACEUTICAL MANUFACTURERS

The pharmaceutical manufacturers have been intensively involved in malaria vaccine research, and to a lesser extent, schistosomiasis. They invest at least $100 million annually in vaccine research, even though few of the vaccines under development affect the major public health problems of the tropics. The research and development efforts have been tempered by the prospects for the size of the market for the potential products. Several drugs for tropical disease have been developed without the involvement of drug companies because the small number of people with the disease or the poverty of those affected, dim the likelihood of financial return on the research investment, for pharmaceutical companies.

5 *Implementation*

Introduction

In 1981, WHO estimated that primary health care could be provided for all with an annual investment of $10 per capita or $30 billion annually between 1980 and 2000 (World Bank, 1987b). The total public and private resources now spent amounts to $13.3 per capita; however, much less is available in the poorest countries (World Bank, 1987b). Since government expenditures may comprise only a small proportion of the total, it is important to assure that these monies are spent in a manner that will most effectively improve health. The cost effectiveness of alternative strategies should also be considered. Decisions on strategies must also account for determinants of health, such as the political situation, community will, and resources available, among other factors. This chapter presents the information currently available on the cost-effectiveness of public health strategies.

Cost-Effectiveness

Value of the Method

Cost-effectiveness analysis serves to compare the costs of alternative strategies to achieve specific health outcomes. The results are generally expressed in terms of lives saved, years of healthy life saved, or immunization coverage. Cost-benefit analysis differs from cost-effectiveness analysis in that it values all outcomes, including lives or years of life and disability, in economic (*e.g.*, dollar) terms. Table 15 presents some results of studies of specific interventions. In some cases, costs of programs were known, but

Table 15.   Cost-Effectiveness of Selected Interventions in Developing Countries (1985 Dollars)

INTERVENTION	ANNUAL COST PER CAPITA ($)	COST PER DEATH AVERTED ($)
EPI (Indonesia)	0.07	210.00
DDT spraying for malaria	3.54	440.00
Oral rehydration therapy (ORT)	0.19	230.00
Home distributed ORT packets (Egypt)	0.63	540.00
Measles vaccination (Ivory Coast)	0.53	850.00
Narangwal primary health care project	3-4.00	300-8000.00
Primary health care projects	1-3.00	?
Education	74.00[1]	2,800.00
Sanitation and water	6-46.00	1,250-19,200
Onchocerciasis Control Program (Upper Volta)		150[2]

1.   Cost per student.

2.   Cost per discounted year of healthy life and per discounted productive year of healthy life added (Prost and Prescott, 1984).

effectiveness was estimated (*i.e.,* malaria, measles vaccine) (Walsh, 1986). From this table it is evident that immunization against the childhood diseases included within the Expanded Programme on Immunization, malaria control in hyperendemic areas, and oral rehydration are the most cost-effective health interventions and a program wishing to avert deaths most efficiently should concentrate on these areas.

Cost-effectiveness analysis can be used to assist public health decision-makers in a variety of ways: (1) it can help program managers compare the benefits of alternative management and organizational strategies; (2) it can aid in making the decision to expand a program from a few demonstration projects to other parts of the country; (3) it can help to decide the merits of continuing a specific program, particularly if the program is funded by foreign assistance that may be temporary; and (4) it can help officials in other countries to predict the cost of undertaking such programs in their own areas and to decide if these costs are justified.

Cost comparisons of alternative strategies for immunization and for the treatment of diarrhea have assisted in making program decisions (Lermer *et al.,* 1985; Shepard *et al.,* 1985; Shepard, *et al.,* 1986; Shepard and Cash, 1984). Creese (1984) calculated that the mean cost per immunization contact in Brazil was about US $4 for vaccines available routinely, on demand, from health centers. The strategy of intensifying routine services by offering the same immunization, with local publicity, administered by health center staff at prearranged outreach clinics in the catchment area of the health center averaged $1.25. Finally, the cost per immunization contact dropped to US $1.10 for a campaign that was heavily publicized and lasted one day only, when immunizations were given by health service staff and workers from other organizations (Creese, 1984; 1986a,b).

A study from Bangladesh compared the cost-effectiveness of three services for the treatment of diarrhea. The services considered were a large "Western-style" treatment center (Matlab), an ambulance service bringing patients to Matlab, and a smaller treatment center staffed by paramedics. Not unexpectedly, the costs per patient and per death averted were many times higher at the centralized, tertiary care hospital than at the decentralized clinic. The average cost per patient was almost four times higher using the ambulance service than the treatment center and five times greater at the Matlab hospital. The average cost per death averted was estimated as US $1300 for the hospital, $357 for the ambulance, and $187 for the local treatment center (Horton and Claquin, 1982).

Deficiencies of the Method

Cost-effectiveness analysis has several inherent difficulties. A detailed analysis requires the collection of an enormous amount of information and may take a substantial period of time. This effort may be shortened through the use of sensitivity analysis, that is, modifying the value of the uncertain parameters within an expected range. This correction permits one to test whether a factor will significantly change the results. For those parameters having the greatest influence on the results, field studies can then be done to determine the value quite precisely.

The achievement of better health can be regarded as a proper goal in its own right. The true social benefits of better health may be underestimated, as many parties aside from the patient may profit. Intersectoral programs improving water supplies, sanitation,

and education, among others, confer enormous additional societal and economic benefits aside from the expected health improvement. For economists, good health is valued in terms of effect on
the productive capacity of a society. Health programs are viewed
as investments in people which enable them to be more productive and to increase their material well-being. In this context, the
question arises: Should a death averted perinatally or among the
elderly be equated with a death averted among the economically
and socially most productive? Ill health may also have subtle
unquantifiable effects not only by decreasing productivity but also
by discouraging innovation and change (Mills and Thomas, 1984).

Primary Health Care

The Narangwal study in Northern India was one of the few
studies that vigorously examined the costs of alternative primary
health care systems and their effects on the health of infants and
children (Kielman, *et al.*, 1983). Most other studies have either concentrated on effectiveness or costs, exclusively, collecting little or
no information on the other (Gwatkin, *et al.*, 1980; Satia, 1983).
Examples of costs of large-scale primary health care projects usually
range from US $1 to $3 per capita annual operating costs. Demonstration and pilot projects, however, tend to cost two to three times
more (Grosse and Plasse, 1984; Robertson, *et al.*, 1984). In the
Narangwal study, the cost per infant death averted by health care
averaged about $144, by nutrition $220, and for nutrition plus
health care $230 (1973 US dollars) (Parker *et al.*, 1978).

Alternatives to Health Services Delivery

• *Education.* Many studies have demonstrated the relationship
between educational level and health. Primary health care may be
cheaper in terms of deaths averted for small-scale pilot projects,
but few large-scale projects have demonstrated direct effects on
deaths averted (Berman, *et al.*, 1986; Chen, 1986; APHA, 1982). In
contrast, the association of lower infant mortality rates and educational level have been obtained from the World Fertility Survey
in addition to smaller scale projects. In this world-wide population-
based survey, many of the confounding variables, such as income
level, could be controlled because of the large numbers of women
involved. The cost-effectiveness of primary health care derives from
actual intervention studies so that a closer causal relationship to
improved health status may be inferred. The relationship between

educational level and health is only an association, however intuitively correct it may seem.

The median costs of education were estimated on the basis of information provided from the World Bank education projects from 1981 to 1983. Annualized capital costs per student to pay for the building (estimated to last 20 years) were US $25; for furnishings (amortized over 5 years) $24; for equipment (amortized over 5 years) $3. The recurrent annual cost for maintenance, utilities, and teacher salaries for a classroom of 30 students was approximately $23 per student. Textbooks were assumed to be purchased by the parents. The family costs not included in this calculation included textbooks, lost wages of the child while in school, expenses for childcare for younger siblings if an older child/caretaker went to school, clothes, extra food, time and expenditures for transport to the school, school fees, and so forth.

According to numerous studies, one year in school for the mother correlates with a decline in the expected infant mortality rate of 9/1000 live births and approximately 5/1000 children (Cochrane, 1986, 1980). However, this putative decline of 9/1000 live births has never actually been tested prospectively. If educated women have on average 3 children a piece, this translates into a cost of approximately $770 per infant and child death averted. Usually, however, a child of 7 to 8 years is sent to school and will have children approximately 15 years later. If the cost is discounted at a rate of 7% for 15 years, then the cost per infant death averted almost trebles. This cost per death averted is higher than that found in primary health care studies, but the calculation only includes one specific health benefit: saving infant and child lives. The same investment in education clearly must benefit the health of other members of the family even though this area has not been studied carefully. In addition, education unquestionably has other societal benefits aside from health improvement.

The mechanism for preventing deaths is unknown and deserves further research. It is independent of socio-economic status and place of residence and probably acts through modifying childcare practices (Caldwell, 1979; United Nations, 1985). Koranic education had only minimal impact on mortality (United Nations, 1985). Certainly in rural areas, diarrheal disease incidence rates are lower among children of educated women. Educated women use family planning methods and have fewer, wider spaced births (Cochrane, 1986). It is unclear whether the content of the school curriculum is the key element, whether it is exposure to peers and peer pressure (for example, learning improved personal hygiene from the teacher and fellow students), or the fact that educated individuals are more likely to change their behavior in response to media messages and health education efforts. The effect of education on health is certainly separate from the higher socio-economic status associated with greater number of years in school. Whether or not the education of children can influence the health of younger siblings is another unknown area.

- *Water Supplies and Sanitation.*   Several studies have demonstrated the impact of water supply and/or excreta disposal improvements on mortality from all causes (Esrey, *et al.*, 1985). The median reduction was 20% with a range of 0-81%. The expected mortality reduction depends upon a number of factors: the present mortality rate, the present status of water and excreta disposal, the incidence of diarrhea and typhoid and their case fatality rates (since provision of water supplies and sanitation has a greater effect on diarrhea and typhoid than on other causes of mortality), the use of the water and excreta facilities, the level of personal hygiene, among others. From the UNDP/World Bank program, the annualized cost in 1982 dollars of urban water supply is $20 for a house connection and $11 for a public tap; for rural water it is $10. For sanitation, the cost is $26 for urban sewerage, $11 for other types of urban disposal facilities, and $4 for rural latrines (Esrey, *et al.*, 1985 quoting UNDP project INT/81/026). More recent World Bank estimates for drilling wells capped with hand pumps are as low as $2 per capita annual cost. These estimates include drilling and maintenance costs, not just the equipment costs. These are most comparable to the costs calculated for provision of immunization or oral rehydration mentioned above which also include not just costs of the vaccine or the ORT solution, but the entire delivery program.

An extraordinarily rough calculation of cost effectiveness in an area with a crude mortality rate of 12/1000, providing both sanitation and water supplies for an annualized cost of $6 per capita for the least expensive rural service would be $1,250 per life saved; for urban service at $46 per capita it would be $19,200. A cost-effectiveness calculation for deaths averted also does not examine the many other non-health benefits of water and sanitation in decreasing the time needed for water drawing on the part of women, releasing this time for other activities (such as mother care, income generation, or family gardening), and improvements in agriculture and animal husbandry from readily available water.

• *Other.* Recently, the WHO, Food and Agricultural Organization (FAO), and United Nations Environmental Programme (UNEP) reviewed the experience on cost-effectiveness using environmental management as a vector control measure (PEEM, 1986). Vector control is known to be both effective and cost-effective in averting deaths, depending on the intensity of vector-borne disease transmission in an area. Environmental management is an alternative that should be considered in efficient planning and management of health resources.

Use of communications and mass media for health promotion has an enormous potential for improving health status. The proportion of the world's population with access to radios and television increases at an incredible rate. Messages can even now be transmitted widely through the use of the stationary satellites. In the future this venue will have an even more powerful influence on individual behavior. Communication and mass media marketing and advertising techniques have been used most extensively and successfully in family planning programs, but examples of other successful uses are: Mexico's program to decrease teenage pregnancy, Brazil's breast-feeding promotion campaign, India's social marketing of contraceptives, Bangladesh's social marketing of oral rehydration, USA's hypertension control program and the program to change sexual behavior of homosexuals, those at greatest risk of transmitting AIDS. UNICEF has spearheaded many of these social marketing and health promotion campaigns in the developing world. No studies have carefully evaluated the cost-effectiveness of communication methods, and particularly the alternative types of media use and educational messages. This is an area requiring study as the potential for increasing use of the media is enormous.

The cost-effectiveness of many potentially quite important interventions is unknown: improved safety measures and their effect on decreasing injuries, the effect of modified cooking stoves on incidence and severity of respiratory infections and burns, measures to decrease the incidence of low birth weight, interventions to improve maternal morbidity and mortality, nutrition.

Cost-effectiveness analysis can be a valuable decision-making tool for weighing alternative strategies for improving health. It does not take into account the many social benefits of interventions which are enormously important, namely, education, water supplies, and excreta disposal. The most cost-effective interventions at present continue to be childhood immunizations and use of oral rehydration for diarrhea. In areas where malaria is endemic, vector control may also be cost-effective. Education and water supplies and excreta disposal are several times more costly per death averted when compared with primary health care, but this calculation does not take into account the additional societal benefits which accrue.

Despite the power of the technique, it is not used widely as few individuals, particularly in the developing world know how to perform such an analysis and apply it locally. Certainly an improvement in this capability among national, regional, and district planners and administrators should result in more efficient management and use of the limited health resources. As part of the District Health program within the Strengthening Health Services Unit of WHO, this deficiency will be addressed. An evaluation of the outcome of this program in terms of its cost-effectiveness may be valuable part of the project.

Implementation Priorities

Fortunately, many of the sicknesses affecting people in the developing world can be treated or prevented. Vaccines, drugs, oral rehydration therapy, health education can shorten days of disability and decrease the risk of dying. Unfortunately, resources are seriously limited and careful planning must take place at all levels to most effectively use those resource to try to improve health equitably. The planning must involve several tiers of complexity: causes of burden of illness, intervention strategies for specific diseases, intersectoral interventions, risk groups, resources available both for health services and for other health-related matters (from governmental and private sector including voluntary organizations, industry and private health workers), among others. Priorities for several of these levels will be discussed separately.

Health Services

• *Disease Specific.* Implementation priorities for specific diseases, distributed through the health services would depend upon the burden of illness in an area but would involve the high priority interventions listed in Table 16. These are inexpensive, efficacious

Table 16. High Priority Interventions—Efficacious, Prevent or Avert a Great Burden of Illness, Inexpensive, Feasible

GLOBAL	ENDEMIC AREAS
Immunization	Malaria Control
Measles ⎤	Schistosomiasis chemotherapy
Whooping Cough ⎥ DTP	Intestinal helminth chemotherapy
Tetanus ⎥	Other immunizations, e.g.,
Diphtheria ⎦	meningococcus
Poliomyelitis	
Oral rehydration	
Antibiotics for pneumonia	
Vitamin A	
Family Planning	

and feasible control measures for diseases causing a great deal of disability and death. Depending on the illnesses prevalent in a particular area, others may be added. These interventions entail:

1.   Immunization for childhood diseases as recommended by the Expanded Programme on Immunization. The efficacy of the BCG vaccine for prevention of pulmonary tuberculosis remains controversial. Thus separate, specific efforts to try to achieve high BCG immunization coverage may not be warranted, but as part of the Expanded Programme on Immunization (EPI) in which the health system is organized to provide a number of immunizations, BCG adds little additional cost. The other components of the EPI are measles, polio, and DTP (diphtheria, tetanus, and pertussis) for children and TT (tetanus toxoid) for pregnant women. When meningococcal meningitis epidemics occur in the endemic areas of sub-Saharan Africa, immunization will prevent transmission of the infection.

2.   Oral Rehydration Therapy for diarrhea.

3.   Acute Respiratory Infection. Even though little information is known about the relative cost-effectiveness of short-term antibiotic treatment for lower respiratory infections, this intervention appears to be relatively inexpensive and efficacious. Pilot studies have demonstrated the efficacy of simplified algorithms for identifying those affected together with the use of short-term antibiotics

in averting childhood deaths from acute lower respiratory tract disease. Results of larger field studies are awaited for evaluating cost-effectiveness and refining treatment methods.

4.   Vitamin A supplementation. Twice-a-year supplements are remarkably inexpensive and easy to distribute. Their use will avert vision impairment from vitamin deficiency and may avert deaths from diarrheal and respiratory disease (Somers, 1986). Several studies of the effect on childhood mortality and morbidity are under way and will help to clarify its role in infant and child health. Prior to publication of the results of these studies, this should be considered a priority.

5.   Family planning. Birth spacing, limiting family size, delaying first pregnancy until after adolescence, and reducing the number of births among women over 35 or 40 will probably have a marked effect on infant and child mortality although this has not yet been examined carefully (Pebley and Millman, 1986).

6.   Malaria control in endemic areas. Through the health services, chemoprophylaxis for infants and pregnant women can be made available in areas where chloroquine resistance is not widespread. Presumptive treatment for clinical disease should occur in a timely fashion. Vector control may not be possible through the health care delivery services but may require other agencies. The cost-effectiveness of vector control methods depends upon the strains prevalent in the area, chemical resistance, and resources available, among other factors.

7.   Health education concerning the importance of personal hygiene. Improved personal hygiene particularly on the part of the household food handler will reduce diarrheal disease incidence (Clemens and Stanton, 1987; Feachem, 1984). Other possible areas for health education include: nutrition, such as appropriate weaning foods, cooking foods more than once a day so that food does not stand at room temperature for long periods risking contamination; and excreta disposal particularly for children. These warrant more limited expenditures of health resources because their efficacy is less well known.

8.   Other specific disease interventions to consider, depending upon the burden of illness locally, include annual or twice yearly chemotherapy for worms and typhoid vaccine if it is available inexpensively.

Health Services Organization

Access to health services has markedly improved, but the impact on health has usually been less than expected. To improve the effectiveness of such services, more attention must be given to the administration, management, planning, evaluation, and information systems used, as well as to encouraging community involvement and political commitment. Evaluation and monitoring systems in the past usually comprised approximately 5% of the health services budget, but a greater investment in this area would probably yield significant returns in augmented effectiveness. Operations research should be an integral function of a health system.

Despite the problems and constraints in the developing world, successful large-scale health and population planning cases can be found. Successful programs have not only reached their stated goals and objectives and demonstrated a measurable health impact, but also have established cost-effective approaches, and many have passed the critical test of sustainability. Success stories can be encountered in the public and private sector, and via both categorical and broadly based approaches. These work largely because people make them work.

There is no magic formula for success that can be universally applied, but there are approaches that are more likely to work in specific situations. Nor can the success of a project or program be separated from the environment, including culture and religion, socio-economic development, equity, socially imposed gender roles, bureaucratic tradition, and political commitment.

Successful case histories in family welfare emphasize good planning with the setting of clear objectives and attainable targets, careful implementation based on a flexible problem-solving approach, a personnel policy that emphasizes training, supervision, and a people-oriented management style, sound financial policies, and continuous monitoring and evaluation. This approach works not only because all of the elements are in place but also because they are sensitive and responsive to carefully studied, situation-specific circumstances, and applied with flexibility and innovation.

Systems work when they respond to people's needs and perceptions, and when people are involved in the planning, implementation, and evaluation. These successes inspire the confidence of the people in their ability to reshape their lives, the confidence of governments that their efforts can make a difference, and the

115

confidence of the international community, that their investments pay off.

In a recent conference sponsored by the Rockefeller Foundation analyzing factors associated with successful, sustained health and family welfare projects, the common elements varied from situation to situation. The following list catalogs all of the factors that have been found in the various programs. Only local conditions can determine which are necessary, but none should be overlooked as potentially important elements of successful population and health programs: (1) financing and at least partial cost recovery, (2) problem-solving approach, (3) public-private interaction, (4) community involvement, (5) management expertise, (6) qualitative and quantitative information systems, (7) training at all levels, (8) use of many types of media for communication, (9) careful policy and planning and strategy consideration, (10) social and political will.

The determination of the elements needed in a particular locale to improve health services requires the sensitive and responsive study of the specific situation to ascertain the people's needs and perceptions.

Health Services Financing.

Fees, particularly for first aid and illness care, do not appear to significantly decrease use of the health care system. When the health care is considered high quality, people are willing to pay. Financing schemes include drug fees, revolving drug funds, fee-for-services, among others (World Bank, 1987b). Fees for illness care may subsidize the preventive health measures, such as immunizations. Financing schemes may require modification to guarantee provision of at least the minimal, most cost-effective interventions mentioned above to those presently underserved and most vulnerable. In areas with several health care sources, the government should consider concentrating on providing only the most cost-effective interventions to the underserved and permit the rest of the population to obtain health care elsewhere, through private voluntary organizations, or other private sources, permitting the government health budget to be appropriated more effectively.

Risk Groups

Those with the worst health status in the population are the poor and the migrants. These groups frequently are the most difficult to reach as they may live in temporary housing and move frequently. They are illiterate, are not members of an established community, and use established services less frequently than others. These individuals comprise the priority group for any health improvement program.

Intersectoral Health-related Activities

The health implications of environmental modification programs, agricultural, and educational programs should be considered at the local, district, regional, and national level. The rapid increase in access to the mass media among people in developing countries is a powerful vehicle for health education. Efforts should be made not only to air specific health education messages but also to integrate health issues into shows, music, stories, movies, serials, etc. The presence of stationary satellites that have the capacity to transmit programs to entire continents simultaneously provides access to a huge audience with relatively little effort and expense. Even though no cost-effectiveness studies are available in this area, the potential for health benefit seems obvious.

Policy Issues

In this arena the UNDP may have an advantage because of its proximity to governments. Political will and commitment to health is an indisputable foundation for health implementation and improvement (Halstead, *et al.*, 1985). The means for stimulating and sustaining commitment will vary from place to place.

Conclusions

Priorities for health improvement exist at a variety of levels. Decisions on which types of programs to select depend on the local situation, economic, political situation, the absorptive capacity, and community will. And once again, setting priorities does not imply exclusivity.

6 *Concluding Remarks*

The United Nations Development Programme, Division for Global and Interregional Programmes generously supported the writing and publication of this monograph in order to further the dialogue amongst the international community about alternatives for health research and services. Traditionally, bilateral and multilateral donors and agencies have accorded relatively little development support to health compared to agriculture or transport or education. Within national budgets, health programs have had no obvious, short-term economic returns (as compared with irrigation, factory building, and electrification). However, there is an increasing realization that health is a key element in quality of life, and health status is an important determinant of economic productivity.

Effective use of the limited resources for health has become even more critical in the 1980's since the world-wide economic recession has placed even greater demands upon the remaining resources. During the past decade the debt burden carried by developing countries has doubled to well over one thousand billion dollars, so that an increasing proportion of the Gross Domestic Product is committed to debt repayment. Health programs have stalled or contracted disproportionately. Health research support stands at the margin of health programs; and therefore has suffered even more severely.

Health research plays an integral part in the health system of every country. When defined broadly as a flexible, problem-solving approach to resolve identified obstacles, it holds the key to overcoming the limitations to raising the quality of life for those most disadvantaged. Research helps to provide the maximum benefit from available resources.

Improvement of well-being requires greater investment in health programs and research and more efficient use of the present resources. Concentration on priorities may promote efficiency; however, if more resources were available, the need for priority-setting would not be so urgent. Several possible approaches to increase resources for health-promoting activities are listed below. A number of these were initially suggested by T. Rothermel, Director for the Division for Global and Interregional Programmes of the United Nations Development Programme at a recent meeting sponsored by The Rockefeller Foundation concerned with health research for the developing world.

1.   Identify population groups with the worst health status and concentrate on providing services for them. These are the poorest and most neglected members of society. Ideally, fee-for-service care and paid health insurance schemes should involve those who have some ability to pay, while public services should reach out to those most deprived (World Bank, 1987b; USAID, 1986).

2.   Encourage and facilitate projects in other sectors (education, agriculture, industry, transport, etc.) which will promote health and limit the detrimental effects of others. For example, an irrigation project may provide more water closer to households and improve agriculture, but it may also increase transmission of schistosomiasis and other water-related diseases. Within the project, a health administrator could try to encourage the establishment of disease prevention efforts, the provision of local clinics to provide care and monitor disease, and education to use the increased water supply for growing small home vegetable patches to improve nutrition. An education or curriculum development project could make use of health topics in its instructional materials. A communication or media program could present health or nutrition

topics on radio or television programs. A plan to open new agricultural areas should include health care services and disease control.

3. Every health project (particularly those internationally funded) should earmark a percentage of the total resources for research. A clear process for setting research priorities and assuring accomplishment of the goals is part of this commitment.

4. New resources for health from taxation of unhealthy products and processes, such as tobacco or toxic chemicals. Such a program may decrease consumption, and the resulting increase in health services and research may avert the toxic effect of these products.

Ministries of Planning, Finance, Health, Agriculture, Industry and others, as well as multilateral, bilateral, and nongovernmental agencies should consider these and other possible innovative ways to increase the visibility of health issues, the political will, and commitment to improved health. Such a commitment would translate into greater resource allocation.

References

American Public Health Association. *Primary health care progress and problems: An analysis of 52 AID-assisted projects.* Washington, D.C., 1982.

Anonymous. Premature mortality in the United States. Public health issues in the use of years of potential life lost. *Morbid Mortal Weekly Report.* 1986;35(2S):1S-11S.

Anonymous. Japanese encephalitis: Report of a World Health Organization Working Group. *Morbid Mortal Weekly Report.* 1984;33:119-25.

Anonymous. Self-reported changes in sexual behaviors among homosexual and bisexual men from the San Francisco City Clinic cohort. *Morbid Mortal Weekly Report.* 1987;36(12):1989.

Arnold RB, Indijati Soewarso T, Karyadi A. Mortality from neonatal tetanus in Indonesia: results of two surveys. *Bull WHO.* 1986; 64(2):259-62.

Ashworth A, Feachem RG. Interventions for the control of diarrhoeal diseases among young children: weaning education. *Bull WHO.* 1985a;63(6):1115-27.

Ashworth A, Feachem RG. Interventions for the control of diarrhoeal diseases among young children: prevention of low birth weight. *Bull WHO.* 1985b;63(1):165-184.

Ashworth A, Feachem RG. Interventions for the control of diarrhoeal diseases among young children. improving lactation. Geneva: WHO. CDD/1985c;2.

Baker SP, Oneill B, Karpf RS. *The Injury Fact Book.* Lexington, Massachusetts: D. C. Heath and Company. 1984

Barnum HN, Barlow R. Modeling Resource Allocation for Child Survival. In: Mosley WH, Chen LC. *Child Survival: Strategies for Research. Population and Development Review.* 1984;10:367-87.

Beasley RP, Lin C-C, Hwang L-Y, *et al.* Hepatocellular carcinoma and hepatitis B virus. A prospective study of 22,707 men in Taiwan. *Lancet.* 1981;ii:1129-33.

Beaton GH, Ghassemi H. Supplementary feeding programs for young children in developing countries. *Am J Clin Nutr.* 1982;35:864-916.

Berggren WL, Ewbank GC, Berggren GG. Reduction of mortality in rural Haiti through a primary health care program. *N Engl J Med.* 1981;304:1224-9.

Berman PA, Gwatkin DR, Burger SE. Community-based health workers: head start or false start towards health for all? Washington, D.C.: World Bank. PHN Technical Note 86-3, January 1986.

Berman S, Duenas A, Bedoya A, Constain V, Leon S, Borrero I, Murphy J. Acute lower respiratory tract illness in Cali, Colombia: A two-year ambulatory study. *Pediatrics.* 1983;71:210-18.

Berman, S, McIntosh K. Acute respiratory infections. In: Walsh JA and Warren KS (Eds.). *Strategies for Primary Health Care: Technologies Appropriate for the Control of Disease in the Developing World.* Chicago: University of Chicago Press, 1986:29-46.

Biswas M, Pinstrup-Andersen P (Eds.). *Nutrition and Development.* Oxford: United Nations University and Oxford University Press, 1985.

Bradley AK, Greenwood AM, Byass P, Greenwood BM, Marsh K, Tulloch S, Hayes R. Bed-nets (mosquito-nets) and morbidity from malaria. *Lancet.* 1986;ii(July 26):204-7.

Bruce-Chwatt LJ. *Essential Malariology.* London: William Heinemann Medical Books Ltd., 1980.

Bulla A. Global review of tuberculosis morbidity and mortality in the world (1961-1971). *World Health Stat Q* 1977;30(1):2-56.

Cairncross S. Low-cost sanitation technology for the control of intestinal helminths. *Parasitology Today.* 1987;3(3):94-8.

Caldwell JC. Education as a factor in mortality decline: an examination of Nigerian data. *Popul Stud.* 1979;33(3).

Cates W, Farley TMM, Rowe PJ. Worldwide patterns of infertility: Is Africa different? *Lancet.* 1985;ii:596-8.

Caskey CT. Disease diagnosis by recombinant DNA methods. *Science* 1987;236:1223-9.

Centers for Disease Control. Center for Prevention Services. Division of Sexually Transmitted Diseases. Proposal Initiative I: Syphilis control during pregnancy in Africa. Sexually Transmitted Disease Technical Support for Prevention, Control, Training and Research in Africa With an Initial Concentration in Kenya: A proposal. January 1986.

Channock RM, Lerner RA (Eds.). *Modern Approaches to Vaccines: Molecular and Chemical Basis of Virus Virulence and Immunogenicity.* New York: Cold Spring Harbor Laboratory, 1985.

Chen LC, Choudhury AKM, Huffman SL. Anthropometric assessment of energy-protein malnutrition and subsequent risk of mortality among preschool aged children. *Am J Clin Nutr.* 1980;33:1836-45.

Clemens JD, Chuong JJH, Feinstein AR. The BCG controversy: A methodological and statistical reappraisal. *JAMA.* 1983;249(17):2362-9.

Clemens JD and Stanton BF. An educational intervention for altering water-sanitation behaviors to reduce childhood diarrhea in urban Bangladesh. I. Application of the case-control method for development of an intervention. *Am J Epidemiol.* 1987;125(2): 284-91.

Cochi SL, Broome CV, Hightower AW. Immunization of US children with *Hemophilus influenzae* type B polysaccharide vaccine. *JAMA.* 1985;253(4):521-9.

Cochrane SH. The effects of education on fertility and mortality. Discussion Paper. Education and training series. Report No. EDT26. Washington, D.C.: World Bank, 1986.

Cochrane SH. The effects of education on health. World Bank. Staff Working Paper No. 405. Washington, D.C.: World Bank, 1980.

Creese AL. Cost effectiveness of potential immunization interventions against diarrhoeal disease. *Soc Sci Med.* 1986a;23(3): 231-40.

Creese AL. The Economic Evaluation of Immunization Programmes: Current Practice and Future Needs. Paper prepared for Task Force for Child Survival Meeting. Centers for Disease Control. Atlanta, 10-11 February, 1986b.

Creese AL. Cost-effectiveness of alternative strategies for poliomyelitis immunization in Brazil. *Rev Infect Dis.* 1984;6(Supplement 2):405-7.

Crompton DWT, Tulley JJ. How much Ascariasis is there in Africa? *Parasitology Today.* 1987;3(4):123-8.

Cvjetanovic B. Health effects and impact of water supply and sanitation. *World Health Stat Q* 1986;39:105-117.

Daniel TM. Tuberculosis. In: Walsh JA, Warren KS (Eds.). *Strategies for Primary Health Care: Technologies Appropriate for the Control of Disease in the Developing World.* Chicago: University of Chicago Press, 1986, pp. 93-106.

Davenport FM. Influenza viruses. In: Evans AS (Ed.). *Viral Infections of Humans: Epidemiology and Control.* New York: Plenum Medical Book Co., 1982, pp. 373-97.

de Ferranti D. Some current methodological issues in health sector and project analysis. Washington, D.C.: World Bank, 1983, PHN Technical Notes GEN 24.

Denny FW and Clyde WA. Acute respiratory tract infections: an overview. *Pediatr Res.* 1983;17:1026-9.

De Zoysa I, Feachem RG. Interventions for the control of diarrhoeal diseases among young children: chemoprophylaxis. *Bull WHO.* 1985a;63(2):295-315.

De Zoysa I, Feachem RG. Interventions for the control of diarrhoeal diseases among young children: rotavirus and cholera immunization. *Bull WHO.* 1985b;63(3):569-83.

Dondero T. EPI target disease surveillance and disease reduction targets. Geneva: WHO EPI/GEN 84/6,1983.

Douglas RM, Kerby-Eaton E (Eds.). *Acute Respiratory Infections in Childhood.* Proceedings of an International Workshop, Sydney, August, 1984. Adelaide, Australia: Department of Community Medicine, 1985.

Doumenge JP, Mott KE. Global distribution of schistosomiasis: CEGET/WHO Atlas. *World Health Stat Q.* 1984;37:168-99.

Drummond MF, Stoddart GL. Principles of economic evaluation of health programmes. *World Health Stat Q.* 1985;38:

Editorial. Acute respiratory infections in under-fives: 15 million deaths a year. *Lancet.* 1985;ii:699-701.

Editorial. Maternal Health in Sub-Saharan Africa. *Lancet.* 1987; i:255-7.

Egemen A, Bertan M. A study of oral rehydration therapy by midwives in a rural area near Ankara. *Bull WHO.* 1980, 58:333-8.

Esrey SA, Feachem RG, Hughes JM. Intervention for the control of diarrhoeal diseases among young children: Improving water supplies and excreta disposal facilities. *Bull WHO.* 1985; 63(4)757-72.

Esrey SA, Habicht J-P. Epidemiologic evidence for health benefits from improved water and sanitation in developing countries. *Epidemiol Rev.* 1986;8:117-28.

EPI Newsletter. *Efficacy of Infant BCG Immunization.* Pan American Health Organization. 1986;7(6):2-3.

Expanded Programme on Immunization, World Health Organization, Geneva. The World Health Organization's Expanded Programme on Immunization: A Global Overview. *World Health Stat Q.* 1985;38:232-52.

Feachem RG. Interventions for the control of diarrhoeal diseases among young children: promotion of personal and domestic hygiene. *Bull WHO.* 1984;62(3)467-76.

Feachem RG. Interventions for the control of diarrhoeal diseases among young children: supplementary feeding programmes. *Bull WHO.* 1983;61(6):967-79.

Feachem RG, Bradley DJ, Garelick H, Mara DD. *Sanitation and Disease Health Aspects of Excreta and Waste Water Management.* New York: John Wiley & Sons, 1983.

Feachem RG, Burns E, Cairncross S, Cronin A, Cross P, Curtis D, Khan MK, Lamb D, Southall H. *Water, Health and Development. London:* Tri-Med Books, Ltd., 1978.

Feachem RG, Hogan RC, Merson MH. Diarrhoeal disease control: reviews of potential interventions. *Bull WHO.* 1982;61(4):637-40

Feachem RG, Koblinsky MA. Interventions for the control of diarrhoeal disease among young children: promotion of breast-feeding. *Bull WHO.* 1984;62(2):271-91.

Feachem RG, Koblinsky MA. Interventions for the control of diarrhoeal diseases among young children: measles immunization. *Bull WHO.* 1983;61(4):641-652.

Field CMB, Connolly JH, Murtagh G, Slattery CM, Turkington EE. Antibiotic treatment of epidemic bronchiolitis—a double blind trial. *Br Med J.* 1975;199:(1):83-5.

Foster A, Kavishe F, Sommer A, Taylor HR. A simple surveillance system for xerophthalmia and childhood corneal ulceration. *Bull WHO.* 1986;64(5):725-8.

Francis DP. Hepatitis B virus and its related diseases. In: Walsh JA, Warren KS (Eds.). *Strategies for Primary Health Care: Technologies Appropriate for the Control of Disease in the Developing World.* Chicago: University of Chicago Press, 1986, pp. 289-298.

Frank O. Infertility in sub-Saharan Africa: estimates and implications. *Pop Dev Rev.* 1983;9:1137-44.

Friedmann PS, Wright DJM. Observations on syphilis in Addis Ababa. 2. Prevalence and natural history. *Brit J Vener Dis.* 1977;53:276-80.

Gallagher SS, Finison K, Guyer B, Goodenough S. The incidence of injuries among 87,000 Massachusetts children and adolescents: Results of the 1980-81 statewide childhood injury prevention program surveillance system. *Am J Public Health.* 1984;74(12): 1340-47.

Gallen ME, Rinehart W. Operations research: lessons for policy and programs. *Popul Rep.* 1986;J(4):814-52.

Germanier R, Furer E. Isolation and characterization of *S. typhi* galE mutant Ty21a: a candidate strain for a live oral typhoid vaccine. *J Infect Dis.* 1975;131:553-8.

Glezen WP, Loda FA, Denny FW. Parainfluenza Viruses. In: Evans AS (Ed.). *Viral Infections of Humans: Epidemiology and Control.* New York: Plenum Medical Book Co., 1982:441-55.

Godal T. In presentation of the 8th Programme Report to the Scientific and Technical Advisory Committee of the Tropical Disease Research Programme, March 1987, Geneva: World Health Organization.

Greenwood B. Acute bacterial meningitis. In: Walsh JA, Warren KS (Eds.). *Strategies for Primary Health Care: Technologies Appropriate for the Control of Disease in the Developing World.* Chicago: University of Chicago Press, 1986:150-67.

Grosse RN, Plasse DJ. Counting the cost of primary health care. *World Health Forum.* 1984;5(3):226-30.

Guan-quing Kan. Tuberculosis control in Beijing. World Health Organization WHO/TB/87. 148, 1987.

Guarner V. Treatment of amebiasis. In: Martinez-Palomo A (Ed.). *Amebiasis.* Amsterdam: Elsevier, 1982:189-213.

Guyatt G, Drummond M, Feeney D, Tugwell P, Stoddart G, Haynes RB, Bennett K, Labelle R. Guidelines for the clinical and economic evaluation of health care technologies. *Soc Sci Med.* 1986;22(4):393-408.

Guyer B, Gallagher SS. An approach to the epidemiology of childhood injuries. Symposium on injuries and injury prevention. *Pediatr Clin North Am.* 1985;32(1):5-15.

Gwaltney JM. Rhinoviruses. In: Evans AS (Ed.). *Viral Infections of Humans: Epidemiology and Control.* New York: Plenum Medical Book Co. Second Edition, 1982:491-519.

Gwatkin DR, Wilcox JR, Wray JD. Can health and nutrition interventions make a difference? Washington DC: Overseas Development Council, 1980.

Hakulinen T, Hansluwka H, Lopez AD, Nakada T. Global and regional mortality patterns by cause of death in 1980. *Int J Epidemiol.* 1986;15(2):226-233.

Halstead S, Walsh JA, Warren KS. *Good Health at Low Cost.* New York: The Rockefeller Foundation. 1985.

Hatcher RA, Guest F, Stewart F, Stewart GK, Trussell J, Cerel S, Cates W. *Contraceptive Technology.* 1986-1987. 13th revised edition. New York: Irvington Publishers, 1986.

Hatton F, Tiret L, Nicaud V. Measurement of accident morbidity. *World Health Stat Q.* 1986; 39(3):268-80.

Henderson RH. In: *Protecting the World's Children.* Task Force for Child Survival Meeting, 1985. New York: The Rockefeller Foundation, 1985.

Henderson RH, Sundarsan T. Cluster sampling to assist immunization coverage: a review of experience with a simplified sampling method. *Bull WHO.* 1982; 60:253-60.

Herz B, Measham AR. The Safe Motherhood initiative: proposals for action. Mimeograph. Washington, D.C.: The World Bank, 1987.

Hewlett EL. Pertussis and Diphtheria. In: Walsh JA, Warren KS (Eds.). *Strategies for Primary Health Care: Technologies Appropriate for the Control of Disease in the Developing World.* Chicago: University of Chicago Press 1986:85-93.

Heymann DL, Floyd VD, Lichnevski M, Maben GK, Mvongo F. Estimation of incidence of poliomyelitis by three survey methods in different regions of the United Republic of Cameroon. *Bull WHO.* 1983;61:501-7.

Hira SK, Ratnam AV, Bhat GJ, *et al.* Congenital syphilis in Lusaka. II. Potential risk and incidence at birth among hospital delivered infants. *E Afr Med J.* 1982a;59:306.

Hira SK, Ratnam AV, Sehgal DB, *et al.* Congenital syphilis in Lusaka. I. Incidence in a general nursery ward. *E Afr Med J.* 1982b;59:241.

Holmes KK (Ed.). *Sexually Transmitted Infections of Man.* New York: McGraw Hill, 1984.

Holmgren J, Lindberg A, Molby R (Eds.). *Development of Vaccines and Drugs against Diarrhea.* 11th Nobel Conference, Stockholm 1985. Lund: Studentlitteratur, 1986.

Horton S, Claquin P. Cost-effectiveness and user characteristics of clinic-based services for the treatment of diarrhea: a case study in Bangladesh. *Soc Sci Med.* 1982;17(11)721-9.

Institute of Medicine. *New Vaccine Development: Establishing Priorities.* Volume I. *Diseases of Importance in the United States.* Washington, D.C.: National Academy Press, 1984.

Institute of Medicine. *Preventing Low Birthweight.* Washington, D.C.: National Academy Press, 1985.

Institute of Medicine. *New Vaccine Development Establishing Priorities.* Volume II. *Diseases of Importance in Developing Countries.* Washington, D.C.: National Academy Press, 1986.

Jordan WS. Impediments to the development of additional vaccines: vaccines against important diseases which will not be available in the next decade. Presented at the International Symposium on Vaccine Development and Utilization. June 9 and 10, 1986. *Rev Inf Dis.* 1988 (in press).

Joy JL. The segments of world population at nutritional risk. *Proc Am Assoc Agric Econ.*, 1980: as quoted in Biswas M, Pinstrup-Andersen P (Eds.). *Nutrition and Development.* Oxford: United Nations University and Oxford University Press. 1985, p. 19.

The Kasongo Project Team. Influence of measles vaccination on survival patterns of seven to thirty-five month-old children in Kasongo, Zaire. *Lancet.* 1981;i:764-7.

Keja K, Chan C, Brenner E, Henderson R. Effectiveness of the expanded programme on immunization. *World Health Stat Q* 1986;39(2):161-70.

Keusch GT, Scrimshaw NS. Control of infection to reduce the prevalence of infantile and childhood malnutrition. In: Walsh JA, Warren KS (Eds.). *Strategies for Primary Health Care: Technologies Appropriate for the Control of Disease in the Developing World.* Chicago: University of Chicago Press, 1986, pp. 298-313.

Kielmann AA, McCord C. Weight-for-age as an index of death in children. *Lancet.* 1978;i:1247-50.

Kielman AA, *et al. Child and Maternal Health Services in Rural India. The Narangwal Experiment. Vol 1, Integrated Nutrition and Health Care.* Baltimore: Johns Hopkins University Press, 1983.

Kuznetsov RL. Malaria control by the application of indoor spraying of residual insecticides in tropical Africa and its impact on community health. *Trop Doc.* 1977;7:81-91

LaForce FM, Lichnevski MS, Keja J, Henderson RH. Clinical survey techniques to estimate prevalence and annual incidence of poliomyelitis in developing countries. *Bull WHO.* 1980; 58:609-20.

Larsson Y, Larsson V. Congenital syphilis in Addis Ababa. *Ethiop Med J.* 1970;8:163.

Lechat MF. Impact of research and technology on the efficiency of primary health care in tropical regions. Report prepared for the Commission of the European Communities. Research Programme "Science and Technology for Development." Contract no. ECI-1310-B 7210-85. 1986.

Lechtig A, Habicht JP, Delgado H, Klein RW, Yarbrough C, Martorell R. Food supplementation during pregnancy, maternal anthropometry, and birth weight in a rural Guatemalan population. *J Trop Pediatr.* 1978;12:212-17.

Lennette EH. Viral respiratory diseases: vaccines and antivirals. *Bull WHO.* 1981; 59(3):305-324.

Leowski J. Mortality from acute respiratory infections in children under 5 years of age: Global estimates. *World Health Stat Q.* 1986;39:138-44.

Lermer SJ, Shepard DS, Cash RA. Cost-effectiveness of the control of diarrheal diseases program in the republic of Indonesia. Harvard Institute for Health Research, Harvard School of Public Health. Mimeographed paper 1986.

Lerner R, Channock RM, Brown F (Eds.). *Vaccines 85: Molecular and Chemical Basis of Resistance of Parasitic, Bacterial, and Viral Diseases.* New York: Cold Spring Harbor Laboratory, 1985.

Mabey DCW, *et al.* Tubal infertility in the Gambia: chlamydial and gonococcal serology in women with tubal occlusion compared with pregnant controls. *Bull WHO.* 1985;63:1107-13.

Malaria Action Programme, World Health Organization, Geneva. World Malaria Situation 1984. *World Health Stat Q.* 1986;39(2): 171-205.

Malison MD, Sekeito P, Henderson PL, Hawkins RV, Okware SI, Jones TS. Estimating health service utilization, immunization coverage, and childhood mortality: a new approach in Uganda. *Bull WHO.* 1987;65(3):325-30.

Manciaux M, Romer CJ. Accidents in children, adolescents and young adults: a major public health problem. *World Health Stat Q* 1986;39(3):227-31.

Martinez-Palomo A. Science for the Third World: An Inside View. *Perspect Biol Med.* 1987;30(4):546-57.

Martorell R. Habicht JP, Yarbrough C, *et al.* Acute morbidity and physical growth in rural Guatemalan children. *Am J Dis Child.* 1975;12:12.

Mata LJ. *The Children of Santa Maria Cauque: A Prospective Field Study of Health and Growth.* Cambridge, MA: MIT Press, 1978.

Mata LJ, Urrutia JJ, Albertzazzie C, *et al.* Influence of recurrent infections on nutrition and growth of children in Guatemala. *Am J Clin Nutr.* 1972;25:1267.

Maurice J, Pearce AM (Eds.). *Tropical Disease Research: A Global Partnership.* Eighth Programme Report: The First Ten Years, with Highlights of the 1985-86 Biennium. Geneva: World Health Organization. 1987.

McDonald EC, Pollitt E, Mueller W, Hsueh AM, Sherwin R. The Bacon Chow study: Maternal nutritional supplementation and birth weight of offspring. *Am J Clin Nutr.* 1981;34:2133-44

McKeown T. *The Modern Rise of Population.* London: Edward Arnold (Publishers) Ltd., 1976.

Meheus A, *et al. Chlamydia trachomatis* in women with acute salpingitis and infertility in Central Africa. In: Oriel D, *et al.* (Eds.). *Chlamydia Infections.* Cambridge: Cambridge University Press, 1986:241-244.

Meheus AZ *et al.* Genital infections in prenatal and family planning attendants in Swaziland. *E Afr Med J.* 1980;57:212.

Merz B. DNA probes promise to transform diagnosis of infectious disease. *JAMA.* 1987 (July 17);258(3):301-2.

Miller LH, Howard RJ, Carter R, Good MF, Nussenzweig V, Nussenzweig RS. Research toward malaria vaccines. *Science.* 1986:(12 Dec);2340;1349-56.

Mills A. Survey and examples of economic evaluation of health programmes in developing countries. *World Health Stat Q* 1985a;38:402-31.

Mills A. Economic evaluation of health programmes: Application of the principles in developing countries. *World Health Stat Q* 1985b;38:368-82.

Mills A, Thomas M. Economic evaluation of health programmes in developing countries. A review and selected annotated bibliography. EPC Publication No. 3, London, London School of Hygiene and Tropical Medicine, 1984.

Monto AS. Coronaviruses. In: Evans AS (Ed.). *Viral Infections of Humans: Epidemiology and Control.* New York: Plenum Medical Book Co. Second Edition, 1982:151-67.

Mora JA, deParedes B, Wanger M, *et al.* Nutritional supplementation and the outcomes of pregnancy. In: Birth weight. *Am J Clin Nutr.* 1979;32:455-62.

Mosley WH. Child survival: Research and policy. In: Mosley WH, Chen LC (Eds.). Child Survival: Strategies for Research. *Popul Dev Rev.* 1984;10:3-23.

Mosley WH, Chen LC. An analytical framework for the study of child survival in developing countries. In: Mosley WH, Chen LC (Eds.). Child Survival: Strategies for Research. *Popul Dev Rev.* 1984;10:25-45.

Muller M. Tobacco and the third world: Tomorrow's Epidemic? London: War on Want. 1978.

Noordeen SK, Lopez Bravo L. The World Leprosy Situation. *World Health Stat Q* 1986;39(2):122-128.

Office of Technology Assessment. Status of biomedical research and related technology for tropical diseases. Washington, D.C.: Congress of the United States. 1985.

Paine PA, Pasquall L, Joaquim MCM. Effects of birthweight and gestational age upon growth in Brazilian infants: a longitudinal study. *J Trop Pediatr.* 1983;29(Feb):11-17.

Pamra SP. Tuberculosis control in India. World Health Organization WHO/TB/87. 1987, p. 149.

Pan American Health Organization. Acute Respiratory Infections in Children. RD 21/1. 1983

Pan American Health Organization. Report of the Ad Hoc Group on Research Policies and Strategies for the Region Towards the Goal of HFA/2000. 1986

Panel of Experts on Environmental Management for Vector Control. Report of the Sixth Meeting. Geneva, 8-12 September, 1986. Geneva: World Health Organization, PEEM Secretariat, 1986.

Parasitic Diseases Programme, World Health Organization, Geneva. Major Parasitic Infections: A Global Review. *World Health Stat Q* 1986;39(2):145-60.

Parker RL, Taylor CE, Kielmann AA, Srinivasa Murthy AK, Uberoi IS. The Narangwal experiment on interactions of nutrition and infections. III. Measurement of services and costs and their relation to outcome. *Ind J Med Res.* 1978;68(Suppl):42-54

Payne D, Grab B, Fontaine RE, *et al.* Impact of control measures on malaria transmission and general mortality. *Bull WHO.* 1976; 54:369-77.

Payne PR. The nature of malnutrition. In: Biswas M, Pinstrup-Andersen (Eds.). *Nutrition and Development.* Oxford: United Nations University and Oxford University Press, 1985:1-19.

Pebley AR, Millman S. Birthspacing and child survival. *Int Fam Plan Perspect.* 1986;12(3):71-79.

Perlman P. Immunogenicity assays for clinical trials of malaria vaccines. *Parasitology Today.* 1986;2(5):127-131.

Petros-Barvazian A and Behar M. Low birth weight—A major global problem. *Ambio.* 1978;7(4):158-63.

Phillips MA, Feachem RG, Mills A. Options for diarrhoea control. The cost and cost-effectiveness of selected interventions for the prevention of diarrhoea. London: Evaluation and Planning Centre for Health Care, London School of Hygiene and Tropical Medicine. EPC Publication No. 13, Spring 1987. ISSN 0267-5994.

Pio A, Leowski J, ten Dam HG. The magnitude of the problem of acute respiratory infections. In: Douglas RM and Kerby-Eaton E (Eds.). *Acute Respiratory Infections in Childhood.* Adelaide, Australia: University of Adelaide, 1985, 3-16.

Poats RM. Twenty-five years of development cooperation: A review. Paris: Organization for Economic Cooperation and Development 1985.

Prentice AM, Watkinson M, Cole TJ, Whitehead RG, Lamb WH. Prenatal dietary supplementation of African women and birth weight. *Lancet.* 1983;ii:489-492.

Preston SH. *Mortality Patterns in National Populations.* New York: Academic Press, 1976.

Proceedings of the DiaTech Workshop. Diagnostics for Use in Developing Countries: I. Typhoid Fever and Diarrheal Diseases. December 5, 1985. Seattle: Program for Appropriate Technology in Health, 1986a.

Proceedings of the DiaTech Workshop. Diagnostics for Use in Developing Countries: II. Malaria. January 8, 1986. Seattle: Program for Appropriate Technology in Health, 1986b.

Proceedings of the DiaTech Workshop. Diagnostics for Use in Developing Countries: III. Technologies for the Rapid Diagnosis of Infectious Diseases. April 8, 1986. Seattle: Program for Appropriate Technology in Health, 1986c.

Prost A, Prescott N. Cost-effectiveness of blindness prevention by the Onchocerciasis Control Programme in Upper Volta. *Bull WHO.* 1984;62(5):795-802.

Puffer RR, Serrano CV. Patterns of Birthweight. Scientific Publication No. 504. Washington, D.C.: Pan American Health Organization, 1987.

Puffer RR, Serrano CV. Patterns of Mortality in Childhood. Washington, D.C.: PAHO Sci Pub. no. 262, 1973.

Quinn TC, Mann JM, Curran JW, Piot P. Aids in Africa: An epidemiologic paradigm. *Science* 1986;234(4779):955-964.

Ratnam AV, Din SN, Chatterjee TK. Sexually transmitted diseases in pregnant women. *Med J Zambia.* 1980;14:75.

Ratnam AV, Din SN, Hira SK, *et al.* Syphilis in pregnant women in Zambia. *Brit J Vener Dis.* 1982;58:355-358.

Reubush TK III, Breman JG, Kaiser RL, Warren M. Malaria. In: Walsh JA, Warren KS (Eds.). *Strategies for Primary Health Care: Technologies Appropriate for the Control of Disease in the Developing World.* Chicago: University of Chicago Press, 1986:47-60.

Rifkin SB, Walt G. Why health improves: Defining the issues concerning "Comprehensive Primary Health Care" and "Selective Primary Health Care." *Soc Sci Med.* 1988 (in press).

Riley I. The aetiology of acute respiratory infections in children in developing countries. In: Douglas RM and Kerby-Eaton E (Eds.). *Acute Respiratory Infection in Childhood.* Adelaide, Australia: University of Adelaide, 1985:33-42.

Riley ID, Alpers MP, Gratten H, Lehmann D, Marshall TF de C, Smith D. Pneumococcal vaccine prevents death from acute lower respiratory tract infections in Papua, New Guinea children. *Lancet.* 1986;ii:877-881.

Rinehart W, Kols A, Moore SH. Healthier mothers and children through family planning. *Population Reports.* 1984;12(3), Series J, Number 27:J659-J696.

Robertson RL, Davis JH, Jobe K. Service volume and other factors affecting the costs of immunizations in the Gambia. *Bull WHO.* 1984;62:729-736.

Rohde JE. Acute diarrhea. In: Walsh JA, Warren KS (Eds.). *Strategies for Primary Health Care: Technologies Appropriate for the Control of Diseases in the Developing World.* Chicago: University of Chicago Press, 1986:14-29.

Romer CJ, Manciaux M. Research and intersectoral cooperation in the field of accidents. *World Health Stat Q.* 1986;39(3):281-284.

Rosero-Bixby L. Infant mortality in Costa Rica: Explaining the recent decline. *Stud Fam Plan.* 1986;17(2):57-65.

Rothenberg RB, Labanov A, Singh LB, Stroh G, Jr. Observations on the application of EPI cluster survey methods for estimating disease incidence. *Bull WHO.* 1985, 63:93-99.

Ross DA. Does training TBAs prevent neonatal tetanus? *Health Pol Plan.* 1986;1(2):89-98.

Rowland MG, Cole TJ. The effect of early glucose-electrolyte therapy on diarrhea and growth in rural Gambian children. *J Trop Pediatr.* 1980;26:54-70.

Rowland MGM, Cole TJ, Whitehead RG. A quantitative study into the role of infection in determining nutritional studies in Gambian children. *Br J Nutr.* 1977;37:441.

Rush D, Stein Z, Susser M. A randomized controlled trial of prenatal nutritional supplementation in New York City. *Pediatrics.* 1980;65:683-697.

Satia JK. Experience in the Indian Family Program with Cost-Effectiveness Analysis. In: Sirageldin I, *et al.* (Eds.) *Evaluating Population Programs; International Experience with Cost-effectiveness Analysis and Cost-benefit Analysis.* New York: St. Martin's Press, 1983:269-318.

Shann F, Barker J, Poore P. Chloramphenicol alone versus chloramphenicol plus penicillin for severe pneumonia in children. *Lancet.* 1985a;ii:684-686.,

Shann F, Gratten M, Germer S, Linnemann V, Hazlett D, Payne R. Aetiology of pneumonia in children in Goroka hospital, Papua, New Guinea. *Lancet.* 1985b;ii:72-85.

Shapiro C, Cook N, Evans D, Willett W, Fajardo I, Koch-Weser D, Bergonzoli G, Bolenos O, Guerrero R, Hennekens CH. A case control study of BCG and childhood tuberculosis in Cali, Colombia. *Int J Epidemiol.* 1985;14(3):441-446.

Shepard DS, Sanoh L, Coffi E. Cost-effectiveness of the expanded programme on immunization in the Ivory Coast: A preliminary assessment. *Soc Sci Med.* 1986;22(3):369-377.

Shepard DS and Cash RA. The cost of an Oral Rehydration Therapy Programme: A Manual for Managers. Mimeographed paper, 1984.

Shepard DS, Brenzel LE, Nemeth KT. Cost-effectiveness of Oral Rehydration Therapy for Diarrheal Disease. 1985 Mimeographed paper prepared for the Division of Population, Health and Nutrition, The World Bank.

Singer B. Mathematical models of infectious diseases: Seeking new tools for planning and evaluating control programs. In: Mosley WH, Chen LC. (Eds.). Child Survival: Strategies for Research. *Popul Dev Rev.* 1984;10:347-365.

Somer A, Tarwotjo I, Djunaedi E, West KP, Lorden AA, Tilden R, Mele L. Impact of vitamin A supplementation on childhood mortality: A randomized controlled community trial. *Lancet.* 1986;ii:1169-1173.

Spieler J. Report of a Joint National Institute of Health (NIH) Agency for International Development (AID)/Program for Applied Research in Fertility Regulation (PARFAR). Workshop on Research and Development of Immunological Methods and Fertility Regulation. *Contraception.* 1985;31:11-29.

Stansfield SK. Acute respiratory infections in the developing world. Strategies for prevention, treatment, and control. *Pediatr Infect Dis J.* 1987;6(7):622-629.

Szmuness W, Alter HJ, Maynard JZ (Eds.). *Viral Hepatitis.* 1981 International Symposium. Philadelphia: The Franklin Institute Press, 1982.

Taket A. Accident mortality in children, adolescents and young adults. *World Health Stat Q* 1986;39(3):232-236.

Taylor CE. The uses of health systems research. Public Health Papers 78. Geneva: World Health Organization, 1984.

Toucher L. Chile: Mortalidad de la 4 anos de edad; tendencias y causas; notas de poblacion. *Revista Latinoamericana de Demografía.* 1981;9(26):27-54.

Tropical Diseases Research. A global partnership. Eighth Programme Report of the UNDP/World Bank/WHO Special Programme for Research and Training in Tropical Diseases, WHO, Geneva, 1987.

Tugwell P, Bennett RJ, Sackett DL, Haynes RB. The measurement iterative loop: a framework for the critical approval of need, benefits and costs of health interventions. *J Chronic Dis* 1986 (in press).

Tursz A. Epidemiological studies of accident morbidity in children and young people: problems of methodology. *World Health Stat Q* 1986;39(3):257-267,

United Nations. Socio-economic differentials in child mortality in developing countries. New York: United Nations, 1985.

United States Agency for International Development. Health Financing Guidelines. Mimeographed paper, 1986.

Viegas DAC, Scott PH, Cole TJ, Eaton P, Needham PG, Wharton BA. Dietary protein energy supplementation of pregnant Asian mothers at Sorrento, Birmingham: during third trimester only. *Br Med J.* 1982;285:592-595.

Villar J, Altobelli L, Kestler E, Belzian J. A health priority for developing countries. The prevention of chronic fetal malnutrition. *Bull WHO.* 1986;64(6):847-851.

Walsh J, Warren KS. Selective Primary Health Care: An Interim Strategy for Disease Control in Developing Countries. *Soc Sci Med.* 1980;14C:145-163.

Walsh JA, Martinez-Palomo A. Control of amebiasis. In: Martinez-Palomo A (Ed). *Amebiasis.* New York: Elsevier 1985, p, 241-261.

Walsh JA. Measles In: Walsh JA, Warren KS (Eds). *Strategies for Primary Health Care: Technologies Appropriate for the Control of Disease in the Developing World.* Chicago: University of Chicago Press 1986:60-72.

Walsh JA. Prioritizing for primary health care: Methods for data collection and analysis. In: Walsh JA, Warren KS (Eds.). *Strategies for Primary Health Care: Technologies Appropriate for the Control of Disease in the Developing World.* Chicago: University of Chicago Press. 1986:1-14.

Walsh JA. The importance of Group B streptococcal infection. *Pediatr Infect Dis.* (1988, in press).

Warren KS. Schistosomiasis. In: Walsh JA, Warren KS (Eds.). *Strategies for Primary Health Care: Technologies Appropriate for the Control of Disease in the Developing World.* Chicago: University of Chicago Press, 1986:72-85.

Watkinson M, Watkinson AM. The impact of domiciliary gluco-electrolyte solution on diarrheal prevelance and growth in children under five years of age in rural West African villages. *Ann Trop Pediatr.* 1982;2:13-16.

Watts T, Larsen SA, Brown ST. A case-control study of stillbirths at a teaching hospital in Zambia, 1979-1980: serological investigations for selected infectious agents. *Bull WHO.* 1984;62:803-808.

Weekly Epidemiological Record. Expanded Programme on Immunization: Use of survey data to supplement disease surveillance 1980;57(47):361-368.

Widy-Wirski R, D'Costa J. Maladies transmises par voie sexuelle dans une population rurale en Centrafrique. In: Rapport, final, 13e Conference technique, pp. 651-654, OECEAC, Yaounde.

Wintemute GJ. Injury mortality and socioeconomic development: An exploratory analysis. *Int J Epidemiol.* 1986; 15(4):540-543.

Wirth DF, Rogers WO, Barker R, Douardo H, Suesband L. Leishmaniasis and Malaria: new tools for epidemiologic analysis. *Science.* 1986;234:975-979.

World Bank. Review of Population, Health, and Nutrition in the Health Sector. Washington, D.C.: World Bank, 1985 (draft).World Bank. World Development Report 1987. Washington D.C., Oxford University Press, 1987a.

World Bank. Financing Health Services in Developing Countries: An Agenda for Reform. Washington, D.C.: World Bank, 1987b.

World Health Organization. Review of Primary Health Care Development. SHS/82.3. 1982a.

World Health Organization. Report of a WHO Scientific Group. Treponemal infections. Technical Report Series 674, Geneva, 1982b.

World Health Organization. National Assessments of Health Care Coverage and of its Effectiveness and Efficiency. Report and Main Lessons of a WHO Collaborative Study. SHS/83.7. 1983.

World Health Organization. The incidence of low birth weight: an update. *Wkly Epidemiol Res.* 1984a;59:205-211.

World Health Organization. A Programme for Controlling Acute Respiratory Infections in Children: Memorandum from a WHO meeting. *Bull WHO.* 1984b;62(1):47-58.

World Health Organization. Case Management of Acute Respiratory Infections in Children in Developing Countries. Report of a Working Group Meeting. Geneva, 3-6 April 1984, WHO/RSD/85.15, Rev.2 1985a.

World Health Organization. Women, Health and Development. A report by the Director-General. 1985. WHO Offset Publication No. 90. 1985b.

World Health Organization. The Control of Schistosomiasis. Report of a WHO Expert Committee. Technical Report Series #782. 1985c.

World Health Organization. Prevention of Maternal Mortality. Report of a WHO Interregional Meeting, Geneva, 11-15 November, 1985. FHE/86.1. 1985d.

World Health Organization. Advisory Committee on Health Research. Health Research Strategy Paper. 1986a.

World Health Organization. Basic Principles for Control of Acute Respiratory Infections. In: Children in Developing Countries. A Joint WHO/UNICEF Statement. 1986b.

World Health Organization. Acute Respiratory Infections. Progress and Current Status of the Programme. Second Report. 1985-6. WHO/RSD/86.30 Rev.1. 1986c.

World Health Organization. Acute Respiratory Infections. A Guide for the planning, implementation, and evaluation of control programmes within primary health care. WHO/RSD/86.29. 1986d.

World Health Organization. BCG Vaccination of the Newborn: Rationale and Guidelines for Country Programmes. Tuberculosis and Respiratory Infections Unit. Division of Communicable Diseases. WHO/TB/86.147 and EPI/GEN/86/10. 1986e.

World Health Organization. Diarrheal Diseases Control Programme. Interim Programme Report 1986. CDD/TAG/87.2, 1986f.

World Health Organization. Proposed Programme Budget for the Financial Period 1988-1989. Geneva: World Health Organization, 1986g.

World Health Organization. Essential Obstetric Functions at First Referral Level. Report of a Technical Working Group. Geneva, 23-27 June 1986. FHE/86.4 1986h.

World Health Organization. Prevention of Maternal Mortality. Report of a WHO Interregional Meeting, Geneva, 11-15 November, 1985. FHE/86.1. 1986i.

World Health Organization-UNICEF. Primary Health Care. Alma Ata Declaration, 1978.

Glossary

ADDR   Applied Diarrheal Disease Research, a program funded by the United States Agency for International Development and administered through the Harvard Institute for International Development.

Adenovirus   One of a group of viruses causing upper respiratory disease and present also in latent infections in normal persons.

Aflatoxin   A toxic factor produced by Aspergillius flavus, a pathogenic mold found on ground nut seedlings, and other crops, responsible for deaths in animals and humans.

African Trypanosomiasis   (see Trypanosomiasis).

AID   United States Agency for International Development.

AIDS   Acquired Immune Deficiency Syndrome.

Alma Ata Declaration   Summary statement of a UNICEF/WHO sponsored meeting in 1978 that has become the foundation for global efforts to increase Primary Health Care. The declaration describes the goals and activities of Primary Health Care.

Ameba   A minute one-cell organism.

Amebiasis   The state of being infected with amebae, especially with *Entamoeba histolytica.*

Antibody   A protein that can specifically combine with another substance (antigen). At least five types exist in the human body: G, M, A, D, and E. Each person has many thousands of antibodies that can combine with a huge variety of substances.

Antigen   This is a substance which by virtue of a particular chemical grouping (an "antigenic determinant") can unite specifically with the combining site of an antibody molecule. An immunogen is a substance that stimulates the body to produce a corresponding antibody. Most antigens also function as immunogens.

Arboviral infections   A group of viruses, including the causative agents of yellow fever, viral encephalitides, and certain febrile infections, such as dengue, which are transmitted to man by various mosquitoes and ticks; those transmitted by ticks are often considered in a separate category (tick-borne viruses).

ARI Acute Respiratory Infections.

Asbestosis Lung disease (pneumoconiosis) caused by inhaling particles of asbestos.

Ascariasis Infection caused by the helminth *Ascaris lumbricoides*. The adult worm usually inhabits the lumen of the intestinal tract. Mild infections are common and asymptomatic but heavy, intense infestations may cause abdominal discomfort, rarely obstruction, and possibly malnutrition.

BCG Abbreviation for Bacillus Calmette-Guérin; a vaccine preparation for the prophylactic inoculation of infants against tuberculosis.

CDC Centers for Disease Control of the United States Public Health Service, Atlanta, Georgia, U.S.A.

CDD Diarrheal Disease Control Programme (a WHO Special Programme).

CHW Community Health Worker.

Campylobacter Recently described gram-negative comma-like organism that produces diarrhea in humans and animals.

CARE Cooperative for American Relief Everywhere. An organization providing development assistance to many countries of the world.

Chemotherapy The treatment of disease by chemical agents; first applied to use of chemicals that affect the causative organism unfavorably but do not harm the patient.

Cholera A name applied to a condition marked primarily by severe watery diarrhea, caused by *Vibrio cholera*.

Ciguaratoxin Toxin found in some fishes in the Caribbean and occasionally in other parts of the world. It can cause flushing, rash, fever, neurological and intestinal symptoms.

Circulatory system The heart, blood vessels, and lymphatic channels for circulating blood and other tissue fluids throughout the body. For the purposes of this monograph, this category of diseases includes cardiovascular diseases and certain degenerative diseases, such as nephritis, cirrhosis of the liver, ulcers of the stomach and duodenum, and diabetes.

Cold chain   System (delivery chain) that ensures refrigerated delivery of heat-labile drugs, pharmaceuticals, vaccines, and other perishables.

Cytomegalovirus   One of a group of highly host-specific viruses that infect many monkeys or rodents with the production of unique large cells bearing intranuclear inclusions. The virus specific for man causes cytomegalic inclusion disease.

DAC   Development Assistance Committee of the OECD. This organization monitors development assistance from its members (most of the Western industrialized countries) to developing countries.

DGIP   Division for Global and Interregional Programmes, of the United Nations Development Programme.

DNA   Deoxyribonucleic Acid.

DOD   Department of Defense of the U. S. Government.

DPT   Diphtheria, Pertussis, Tetanus Vaccine also sometimes referred to as DTP.

DTP   (see DPT.)

Dengue   Disease caused by one of the four types of dengue viruses. The usual symptoms are fever and bone pain lasting 5-7 days. However, the majority of infections are asymptomatic. A small percentage of infected young people develop Dengue Hemorrhagic Fever and Shock Syndrome, which carries a high risk of death. It is transmitted by the Aedes mosquito.

Diarrhea   Bowel movements that occur more frequently than usual (*e.g.*, more than 5 times daily) and have a more liquid consistency than usual.

DIATech   Diagnostic Technology for Community Health. A program funded by the USAID to develop and distribute technologically appropriate diagnostic tests for the developing world.

Diphtheria   Disease caused by *Corynebacterium diphtheriae*. Nasopharyngeal infection with the organism produces a toxin which can cause severe local edema, cardiac and skeletal muscle destruction, and nervous system disease. The disease can be prevented by immunization with the inactivated toxoid in DPT vaccine.

Difluoromethyl ornithine   New drug for African trypanosomiasis presently undergoing clinical trials.

Drancunculiasis   Infection with *Dracunculus medinensis* (guinea worm). The female parasite attacks the feet and legs of those standing in water. It pierces the skin and connective tissue and grows slowly over a year to approximately a meter in length. This results in disabling wounds over the legs. A fresh water snail *Cyclops quadricornus* serves as intermediate host.

Enteroviruses   Intestinal viruses, only a small proportion of which produce disease.

Endemic   (1) Present in a community at all times, but occurring in only small numbers of cases. (2) A disease of low morbidity that is constantly present in a human community.

Enterotoxigenic   Producing or containing a toxin specific for the cells of the intestinal mucosa.

EPI   Expanded Programme on Immunization of the World Health Organization.

E. coli   (Escherichia) a species of organisms constituting the greater part of the intestinal flora of man and other animals.

Excreta   Waste matter excreted by the body as urine or feces.

FAO   Food and Agriculture Organization.

Filariasis   A diseased state due to the presence of filariae (a nematode worm) within the body.

GND   Great Neglected Diseases. A program of the Rockefeller Foundation to fund and stimulate research on tropical diseases.

Giardiasis   Infection with Giardia. A genus of flagellate protozoal organisms found in the intestinal tract of man and animals, but not known to be pathogenic, although infection by it is frequently accompanied by a severe diarrhea.

HBsAg   Hepatitis B Surface Antigen.

HIV   Human Immunodeficiency Virus. The virus that produces AIDS.

HRP   Human Reproduction Programme of the World Health Organization.

Helminth   A worm or worm-like parasite.

Hepatitis A   (see hepatitis B virus.)

Hepatitis B Virus   The etiological agent of viral hepatitis. Several types are recognized: (1) hepatitis virus A, the agent causing infectious hepatitis, acquired by parenteral inoculation or ingestion, and (2) hepatitis B, the agent causing serum hepatitis, transmitted by inadequately sterilized syringes and needles, or through infectious blood plasma, or certain blood products. Hepatocellular carcinoma develops in some of the long-term carriers of the virus. (3) Non-A, non-B hepatitis is probably caused by at least 2 separate viruses.

Herpes   An inflammatory skin disease characterized by the formation of small vesicles in clusters. As commonly used, the term alone refers to herpes simplex.

Hookworm   Infection with the helminth *Necator americanus* or *Ancyclostoma duodenale.* The adult worm inhabits the small intestine where it attaches to the epithelium and lives on blood. Intense infestations result in anemia, mild infestations are asymptomatic. Eggs are excreted in the feces and infection is transmitted by walking barefoot on fecally contaminated soil.

Human Immunodeficiency Virus   (see HIV.)

ICDDR,B   International Centre for Diarrheal Disease Research, Bangladesh.

IDRC   Canadian International Development Research Center.

IOM   Institute of Medicine. Part of the United States National Academy of Sciences.

IUGR   Intrauterine Growth Retardation.

Injuries   Damage; wound; trauma. This category includes illnesses resulting from burns, motor vehicle accidents, falls, and occupational accidents or exposures among others.

Intersectoral analysis   Involving other sectors of societies besides health, *e.g.,* education, agriculture, economic, transport, etc.

Immunogenicity   Immunogenic, producing immunity.

Ivermectin   New drug effectively treating onchocerciasis (river blindness).

Japanese B encephalitis   Viral infection found in some parts of Japan and China that can result in paramount disablement. It is transmitted by the Aedes mosquito.

Legionella   Bacterial pathogen initially described in the mid 1970's. Usually it produces a pneumonia but infection with some species only induces a febrile illness.

Leishmaniasis   A disease caused by Leishmania, a genus of flagellate protozoa, parasitic in the human and animal bodies. The Leishmania are found as small oval or round intracellular organisms, chiefly in the reticuloendothelial cells of the skin or the viscera. In the phlebotomine (sand fly) insect host they develop into slender, elongated, nucleated organisms (leptomonad stage). Various species of Leishmania are endemic in many parts of the developing world. The disease causes skin lesions that usually heal slowly, but in a small percentage of individuals, facial destruction or systemic diseases can occur.

Leprosy   A chronic communicable disease, caused by a specific microorganism, the *Mycobacterium leprae* which produces various granulomatous lesions in the skin, the mucous membranes, and the peripheral nervous system. Two clinical types are recognized: (1) cutaneous, lepromatous, or nodular, and (2) neural or maculo-anesthetic. A combination of these types is called mixed leprosy.

Low Birth Weight   Less than 2,500 grams weight at birth. The most important determining factor of survival and quality of life is condition of the child at birth. Those children born with low birth weight have an enormously greater risk of death in infancy and childhood and of disablement throughout life.

Malaria   An infectious febrile disease caused by protozoa of the genus Plasmodium which are transmitted by mosquitoes. Characterized by attacks of chills, fever, and sweating.

Malnutrition   A state in which the physical function of an individual is impaired to the point where he or she can no longer maintain an adequate level of performance. This state results from inadequate nutrition and not from any other known disease process.

Maternal mortality   Death of a woman during pregnancy, delivery, or within one month following delivery.

Measles   A highly contagious parvovirus infection. Infection causes 7-10 days of fever, rash, sore eyes, cough and diarrhea. Secondary complications are frequent, such as pneumonia, ear infections, excess weight loss, and malnutrition. The vaccine is 95% protective.

Mefloquine   New antimalarial drug that effectively treats most chloroquine-resistant malaria.

Meningitis   Bacterial infection of the tissues covering the brain. Untreated, it is uniformly fatal; however, even with antibiotic treatment, 20% or more may die and others suffer chronic neurologic disability.

Mycoplasma   A taxonomic name given a genus including the pleuropneumonia-like organisms (PPLO) and separated into 15 species on the basis of source, glucose fermentation, and growth on agar media. It causes pneumonia in children and adults, and genital infections.

NIH   National Institutes of Health (U.S.).

Neisseria gonorrhoeae   Specific etiologic agent of gonorrhea.

Neoplasm   A focus of progressive, uncontrolled new tissue growth. The growth or tumor may manifest varying degrees of autonomy. Commonly called cancer. The neoplasm may be invasive (malignant) or benign.

OECD   Organization for Economic Cooperation and Development.

OTA   Office of Technology Assessment of the United States Congress.

Onchocerciasis   Infection with the filaria *Onchocerca volvulus*. Intense infection leads to progressive itchy dermatitis and blindness.

PATH   Program for Appropriate Technology in Health primarily funded through the USAID.

PRICOR   Primary Health Care Operations Research. A program funded by USAID to support operations research. Its office is in Chevy Chase, Maryland.

Pathogen   Any microorganism or other substance causing disease.

Periphery   Outskirts of main population centers, usually rural areas having low population density.

Pertussis   (see Whooping Cough)

Picorna viruses   Picornavirus. A name applied to one of the extremely small ether-resistant ribonucleic acid viruses, the group comprising the enteroviruses and the coryonaviruses.

Plasmodium falciparum The species which causes estivo-autumnal malaria in man. It is characterized by the "signet-ring" forms of trophozoites and the "crescent" form of the gametes.

Plasmodium vivax Species causing benign tertian form of malaria.

Poliomyelitis Diseases caused by the poliovirus. Paralysis results from about one percent of infections—most infections are asymptomatic. The oral live attenuated or injectable, inactivated vaccine prevents more than 95% of infections.

Praziquantal Drug for treatment of schistosomiasis. It has remarkably few side effects.

Protozoan (pl.) protozoa. A primitive organism consisting of a single cell.

Quinghaosu Chinese herb and effective antimalarial drug.

RNA Ribonucleic Acid.

Rabies Infection caused by the rabies virus. It is uniformly fatal in man and transmitted from animals by the bite of a carnivore (dog, cat, bats, etc.).

Reactogenicity The ability of vaccines or other drugs to produce side effects or reactions.

Reduviid Belonging to the family Reduviidae and the vector of American trypanosomiasis (Chagas' Disease).

Reduviidae A family of winged hemipteros insects called conenose bugs, kissing bugs, and assassin bugs because they prey on other insects. The vector of Chagas Disease.

Respiratory diseases Acute and chronic illnesses affecting any part of the respiratory tract including nose, tonsils, pharynx, ears, bronchi and lungs. These diseases can be caused by a variety of pathogens and toxins.

Rheumatic Fever and Heart Disease Rheumatism involves a variety of disorders marked by inflammation, degeneration, or metabolic derangement of the connective tissues. In heart disease, it is involvement of the heart by the rheumatic fever process.

Rotavirus Viral pathogen of diarrheal disease particularly in children.

Salmonella spp A genus of microorganisms of tribe Salmonelleae, family Enterobacteriaceae, order Eubacteriales, consisting of rod-shaped, gram-negative bacteria. *S. typhosa* is the etiologic agent of typhoid fever. Most other species of *Salmonella* produce a self-limited diarrheal disease. However, a small number of species can produce a typhoid-like illness (*S. paratyphoid, S. cholerasuis, S. typimurium*).

Schistosomiasis The state of being infected with flukes of the genus Schistosoma.

Shigella spp A genus of microorganisms of tribe Salmonelleae, family Enterobacteriaceae, order Eubacteriales, consisting of non-motile, rod-shaped, gram-negative bacteria. Microorganisms which cause dysentery.

South American Trypanosomiasis (see Trypanosomiasis).

Staphylococcus A spherical bacterium occurring predominantly in irregular grape-like clusters of cells as a consequence of failure of the daughter cells to separate following cell division. It usually causes superficial abscesses; however, occasionally it can produce febrile illness with an erythematous rash called "toxic shock".

Streptococcus A genus of microorganisms of the tribe Streptococ-ceae, family Lactobacillaceae, order Eubacteriales. The beta-hemolytic group represents the human and animal pathogens, alpha-hemolytic group (parasitic) exist as normal flora in upper respiratory tract and intestine. Group A streptococcus sometimes causes an infection in the pharynx and rheumatic fever. Other types of Group A streptococcus can rarely cause a renal disease, acute glomerulonephritis. Group B streptococcus causes disease in pregnant women and newborns.

Syphilis Disease caused by *Treponema palladum*. A chronic sexually transmitted disease causing genital ulcers and many years later, without treatment, cardiac, skin, and cerebral manifestations occur. Syphilis in pregnant women results in pregnancy loss, low-birth-weight infants, and disabling congenital syphilis.

TT Tetanus Toxoid for pregnant women.

TDR World Health Organization's Special Programme for Tropical Disease Research.

Tetanus Disease caused by toxin produced by the bacteria *Clostridium tetani*. It is characterized by painful tonic muscular contractions and is at least 50% fatal if untreated. It is prevented by vaccination with the inactivated tetanus toxoid either alone or given with DPT.

Trachoma A chlamydial disease of the conjunctiva and cornea, producing photophobia, pain, lacrimation, and characterized by pannus and by redness and inflammation. Recurrent and/or persistent trachoma can cause blindness.

Trichuriasis Infection with the intestinal helminth *Trichuris trichiura* (whipworm). Infection is usually asymptomatic but intense infection can cause bloody diarrhea, anorexia, and edema.

Trypanosomiasis A disease caused by the protozoa Trypanosoma. In man it causes sleeping sickness (African Trypanosomiasis) or cardiac failure (Chagas' disease or South American Trypanosomiasis). It is transmitted from animal-to-man or man-to-man by the reduviid bug in South America and the tsetse fly in Africa.

Tuberculosis An infectious disease caused by *Mycobacterium tuberculosis*, and characterized by the formation of tubercles in the tissues. One of the most common chronic respiratory diseases in the developing world.

Typhoid A disease caused by *Salmonella typhosa* and marked by malaise, severe headache, sustained high fever, and occasionally a macular eruption.

UNDP United Nations Development Programme.

UNEP United National Environmental Programme.

UNICEF United Nations International Children's Emergency Fund.

USA United States of America.

USAID United States Agency for International Development.

Vaccinia Virus comprising the smallpox vaccine.

Vector Refers to an agent that transmits a disease, such as insects, including mosquitoes.

Viruses   One of a group of minute infectious agents, characterized by a lack of independent metabolism and the ability to replicate only within live host cells. Individual particle consists of nucleic acid, either DNA or RNA, but not both, contained within a protein coat. If classifed according to origin: reoviruses, if by mode of transmission: arboviruses or tick viruses, if by the manifestations they produce: polioviruses, polyoma viruses, poxviruses.

Whooping Cough   Infection by the bacteria *Bordetella pertussis* and also caused by pertussis. Disease is manifested by prolonged cough with a characteristic inspiratory whoop at the end of a cough spasm. Over 80% of cases are prevented by appropriate vaccination, but 3 doses of DPT are needed.

WHO   World Health Organization.

Yellow Fever   Infection caused by a virus transmitted by mosquito. In its full-blown form the disease presents with fever, jaundice, and bleeding. *Aedes aegypti* transmits the infection in endemic areas of Africa and the Americas. The vaccine can prevent 90% of the cases.

Zoonosis   (pl.) zoonoses. A disease of animals that may secondarily be transmitted to man.